A
Long
Journey Back

Chris R. Pownall

PNEUMA SPRINGS PUBLISHING UK

First Published in 2011 by:
Pneuma Springs Publishing

A Long Journey Back
Copyright © 2011   Chris R. Pownall

Chris R. Pownall has asserted his right under the
Copyright, Designs and Patents Act, 1988, to be
identified as Author of this Work

Pneuma Springs

British Library Cataloguing in Publication Data

Pownall, Chris R.
  A long journey back.
  1. Pownall, Rob--Health. 2. Head--Wounds and injuries--
  Patients--Biography. 3. Paralytics--Great Britain--
  Biography.
  I. Title
  362.1'9751'0092-dc23

  ISBN-13: 9781907728280

Pneuma Springs Publishing
A Subsidiary of Pneuma Springs Ltd.
7 Groveherst Road, Dartford Kent, DA1 5JD.
E: admin@pneumasprings.co.uk
W: www.pneumasprings.co.uk

A
Long
Journey Back

True-life story of Rob Pownall's near fatal head injury
and the battle to regain his life

ACKNOWLEDGEMENTS

I wish to extend my grateful thanks to the following individuals who have kindly assisted in some of the research and preparation for this book: -

- Mr Palitha S. Dias FRCS (England) FRCS (Surg Neurol)
- Judith Mitchell (The Royal College of Surgeons)
- Robert Pownall
- Tracey Kirk
- Patricia Ann Pownall

FOREWORD

This is the real life story about Rob Pownall's near fatal head injury. The accident happened in 1990 when Rob was 18 years old. The story describes his family situation at the time of the accident. It goes on to detail events thereafter, including his life saving surgery, time spent in a coma, and the long journey back to recovery.

When Rob woke up from his coma, he was completely paralysed and had to learn how to speak, and regain the use of his body. Rob has excellent recall of what it was like to be lying in a coma, being aware of what's going on around him, but unable to move a muscle, or communicate with the outside world. The book describes Rob's courage and determination to get his life back, plus all the superb medical treatment and care administered by the NHS (National Health Service).

This account details the care provided by his mother Pat and the effects upon family life, including his older sister Tracey, and me, Rob's father. Although it is has been written by me, there is a chapter which details Rob's recollections of the whole experience, both at the time of the accident, and thereafter.

This book is intended to be an inspiration to others who might find themselves in a similar situation, and need something to give them hope and courage. It's easy to be negative, lose hope and slump into despair and self pity, but Rob remained mentally strong, and maintained a positive mental attitude that was to help him back from what first appeared to be a hopeless and impossible situation.

In view of the fact that some parts of this story are more than a little sad, and have proved difficult for me to relate, the book includes a chapter that contains humorous stories, based upon Rob's wicked sense of humour.

I do hope you appreciate the story of Rob's near fatal head injury and the part played by the NHS in bringing him back from the brink of death. We all hear a lot of bad publicity about our National Health Service; this book provides an opportunity for Rob and I to show another side of the NHS, by detailing the sterling care and services provided by the medical teams of four hospitals in the Sheffield area.

1

The Accident

It was the year 1990, we were living in the North Nottinghamshire town of Worksop, life was good for the Pownall family comprising me Chris, my wife Pat, our daughter Tracey and of course, our son Rob. At the time Pat had recently gained promotion in her work, and this meant that we could afford those little luxuries, which make all the difference to every day living. Tracey had a good job working for a high street bank in the nearby village of Bawtry, and Rob was working for a DIY store in Worksop, until something with better career prospects came along.

Both Rob and Tracey had achieved good 'A' level results, but neither wished to go to university. Rob had worked hard to pass three 'A' levels in Economics, Modular Technology and General Studies. Both Tracey and Rob were driving smart new cars, and we seemed to be progressing nicely, on all fronts. Our cosy lives were about to be interrupted but we did not know it. Then it happened; Robert Pownall, known to his family and friends as Rob had an unfortunate accident that resulted in a near fatal head injury.

Rob is our second offspring, born in May 1972. He was eighteen years of age at the time of his accident, and he was doing just fine. He had worked part time for the Great Mills DIY store whilst he was studying for his 'A' levels, and they kindly offered him full time employment, once his studies were completed. Pat and I were very proud of both our children, particularly in respect of how readily they had adapted to being re-located twice during their years of state education. My work had taken us from Leek in Staffordshire, to Syston in Leicestershire, and then in 1982, we moved to Worksop. They had settled into their new environments, and respective schools, and now both of them had a good circle of friends, here in Worksop.

Looking back, it's amazing how quickly your family grow up particularly when you are enjoying yourselves. In the early days we had mainly camping holidays, which included some of the most memorable ones. We discovered a small campsite in North Wales, located in a small village named Tydweiliog. It was owned by Mr and Mrs Griffith who we got to know extremely well. They became good friends, and that made our holidays even more special. We called Mr John Griffith, Farmer Johnnie, as he ran a smallholding, in addition to the campsite. He had some pedigree sheep that he exhibited at local shows, plus a few chickens, which provided them with eggs for their own consumption, as well for selling on to locals in the village. In addition, Farmer Johnnie had a full time job on a nearby estate, where he was gardener, and general handy man. He was very religious, and on Sundays, he ran the children's Sunday school at the nearby Chapel. He thought the world of the children that regularly visited the campsite, and he would go out of his way to entertain them. I remember one Sunday evening in mid-summer, when he hitched up a trailer to his Massey Ferguson tractor, and gave Tracey and Robert a ride round the field, whilst they sat in the trailer.

We had a number of family holidays abroad, including a trip to Disney World Florida. Naturally, by the time 1990 came along, both Tracey and Rob were becoming independent regarding holidays, and wished to do things on their own.

We had a number of pet dogs whilst the children were growing up, the first being Rusty, a Pembrokeshire Corgi. He was a nice looking dog but he was very destructive, and caused us a lot of damage. When he was about five years old, he became very aggressive, and regrettably, he had to be put to sleep. The vet thought he had developed a brain tumour. Shortly after this, the family moved to Leicestershire, and we acquired Reggie, he was a longhaired Dachshund, a handsome little chap, but unfortunately, he had a bad temper. He was OK with Pat and the children, but on occasion, he would give me the odd nip. We unfortunately lost Reggie, when he was about five years of age, again, due to a terminal illness. The family was very upset at the sad loss of Reggie, so whilst out doing my work, I called in to an animal rescue centre to see what they might have. We had paid a lot of money for our pedigree dogs, and neither had reached a full life span. I walked along the row of kennels, and there was a Border Collie cross bitch, sat with her paw poking through the wire mesh door. I bent down and grasped her paw, and said, "You're a friendly little dog". I asked the person in charge if I could bring the family along in the evening, to see what they thought. As we arrived at the rescue centre, I told Pat and the children I had seen a dog that I liked the look of, but they had to decide. We walked along the row of kennels, and both Tracey and Rob made a beeline for the Border Collie bitch. She was only nine months old, and we christened her Flossy. She was a lovely dog, and we all thought the world of her. She was there whilst the children were growing up, and she enjoyed many holidays at Tydweiliog.

They say that trouble in life occurs when you are least expecting it, and that was certainly true in our case. It was a Friday evening, the 12th of October 1990, and Pat and I were relaxing at home, following another busy week at work. As usual on a Friday evening, Tracey and Robert had gone out with friends; Tracey in her new Nissan Micra and Robert on foot, as no doubt he would be having a drink or two, with his mates in Worksop town centre. This was a regular Friday evening occurrence, long before the age of binge drinking, and Rob assumed responsibility for his conduct, when socialising with his friends.

Friday night was relaxation time for Pat and I, as we were both working extremely hard, and the weekends were something we both looked forward to. I was travelling many miles each week; working for James Walker & Co Ltd, an international engineering manufacturing company. Pat had to be at the bakery shop in Worksop before 07.00am for each of four weekday mornings, so when Friday night arrived, we were both generally quite tired, and in need of some rest. As usual, we had a pleasant evening; I guess, quietly reflecting on things in general, before retiring to our bed at about 10-30pm. Pat would be at the shop early the following morning, so a late night was not for us. Typical of any Friday evening, we would relax after dinner with a few drinks, and maybe, watch a bit of television. It was probably the only night of the week when Pat and I would have the house to ourselves, and although we loved our teenage offspring dearly, the peace and quite from music systems turned off, made a very nice change. It was also the one night of the week when there was no queuing for the bathroom. We had more arguments than enough about access to the bathroom, mainly resulting from Tracey, seemingly being in there for ages.

Once the children had gone out on a Friday evening, Pat and I could have a relaxing bath, with no banging on the door from either Rob or Tracey, shouting, "Father, get yourself out of there quick, I'm going to be late." Now nicely relaxed after a busy day, we were tucked up in bed ready for a good night's rest.

We had both dropped into a deep sleep, when I was awakened by the shrilling tone from our bedside telephone. You know what it's like when you are startled by the phone ringing, and not fully with it when you put the receiver to your ear. It was one of Rob's friends on the line, a nice lad by the name of Andy Sumpter. He said I should not be concerned, but unfortunately, Rob had been involved in an accident, and he was now receiving treatment at the nearby Bassetlaw District Hospital. He said Rob had fallen down and banged his head, whilst returning from an evening in Worksop town centre. Andy explained that he had informed two nearby policemen, who arranged for an ambulance to take Rob to hospital. He said that Rob had suffered no serious injuries, but they were keeping him in hospital overnight, purely as a precaution, and there was no need for me to worry, or to attend the hospital. All being well, Rob would be coming home the next morning.

Pat was now awake, and after I had broken the news to her, we lay there in a state of shock, pondering what might have happened. We wondered if he had been involved in some kind of disturbance, or perhaps a fight. You think all manner of things, when given that type of information. It takes you a minute of two to pull yourself together, when you receive unexpected news like that. We both knew that Andy was a sensible lad, but my fatherly instincts told me that I should get to the hospital straight away. At least I could assess the situation first hand, and hopefully, that would put our minds at rest. Having had a few beers during the course of the evening, I had to get to the hospital on foot. It was no more than a mile from where we lived at the time, so I was there in less than ten minutes. I remember running a bit, and then walking a little, until I had got my breath back. It reminded me of when I was a young lad in Cheshire, and I had to walk along a road lined with sycamore trees, to catch my bus. Very often, I would be late, so to catch up, I would walk the distance between two trees, and then run the next one. That way, you get the chance to recover your breath, before the following run. Having said that, I do remember puffing, and panting by the time I arrived at the hospital. I was now forty-seven years of age, and that run a bit, and then walk a little, was not working as well as it did when I was a lad.

I had never attended an A & E hospital at that time of night, and was shocked to find that all the entrances were securely locked. I couldn't believe this, and had to ring a bell before someone came, to allow me access. I hadn't realised that some hospitals were experiencing major security issues at night, mainly from individuals, under the influence of drink or drugs. I remember thinking, this can't be right, and what ever is the world coming to. I was shown into a side ward within the A & E department, where Rob lay on a trolley, in one of those curtain-partitioned cubicles. He looked in a very bad way to me, but I was assured, both by an attending nurse, and a young A & E doctor, that he would be fine. It was absolutely manic in that department, with people shouting, and the poor staff, were rushed off their feet. The doctor told me he was trying to treat a man, who claimed he had drank at least a full bottle of vodka, as well as numerous pints of beer. It was apparent that all those being treated that night, including Rob, had in one way or another, been involved in an incident, that was in someway, associated with the drinking of alcohol. The doctor told me he didn't believe Rob was drunk, when he was admitted to the A & E department, and I suppose Rob's mate Andy, would have confirmed that they had each consumed a few beers, during the course of the evening.

Rob was incoherent, and I couldn't get any response from him whatsoever. He just lay there with a paper bowl in front of him, as he had been rather sickly; they said this was caused by a bang to his head, rather than the booze. He looked very pale, and whilst his eyes were open, he was apparently unconscious. He lay on his back simply staring at the ceiling, and it appeared to me, that although his eyes were open, the lights were out. They explained that his condition was due to concussion, but I wasn't convinced. I sat at his side, and the nurse kept peering into his left ear, trying to detect where a steady trickle of blood was coming from. She couldn't find any cuts or grazes to explain the source of the blood, and it was obvious to me, that he was bleeding from within his inner ear. Other than the blood seeping from his left ear, there was no sign of any superficial injury, resulting from his accident. I then noticed that his eyes were glazing over, and each eye was looking in a different, and opposed direction. This made him look very strange, and unsightly, from how he appeared normally. I couldn't get my head round why a knock on the head, should have distorted his vision to such a degree; it just didn't make any sense. Had there been a large wound on his head, it would have been more plausible. I would have expected him to have regained consciousness by now, if all he had suffered, was a knock out blow. We have all seen boxers knocked unconscious in the ring, but usually, within a few seconds, they recover, and although a bit unstable, they are up on their feet. Having said that, we are all aware that occasionally, boxers have suffered a severe haemorrhage from being knocked out, and some have not survived.

It all seemed very scary to me, seeing him like that was not pleasant, and I was convinced that something was seriously wrong inside his head. I asked to see the doctor again, and I told him that I thought Rob was very badly injured, and feared that his life was slipping away. He tried to reassure me that there was nothing seriously wrong, but said he would send Rob for an x-ray on his head. It seemed like an eternity, as I sat there waiting and fearing the worst. I had never seen anyone with vision distortion like that, and to me; it was a very bad sign. I had heard about the effects of concussion, but these seemed extreme symptoms to me.

Some five or ten minutes later, Rob was returned to the cubicle, and by now, it was obvious that he was deteriorating fast. It just appeared that he was slipping away, and there didn't seem to be any real sense of urgency. I expressed my growing concern to the nurse, and she began tickling the bottom of both Rob's feet, but she was unable to get even a hint of response. I could see now that she too was becoming concerned, and then the doctor appeared once more. I guess by now he had seen the x-ray results, and a state of emergency, bordering on to panic, had set in. There was a discussion between the doctor and nurse away from my earshot, and then the doctor made a lengthy telephone call, after which he asked me to take a seat. He explained that Rob was suffering from some type of intercranial haemorrhage, and that an emergency ambulance would be transferring him to the Royal Hallamshire Hospital, in Sheffield, where upon, he would undergo immediate surgery. He said a doctor would be travelling with him in the ambulance, and there would be a surgeon at the Royal Hallamshre Hospital, on standby, and all prepared, by the time the ambulance arrived at the Head Injury Unit. He told me that I would not be allowed to travel in the ambulance with Rob, in case they needed to carry out open chest heart massage, whilst the ambulance was in transit. I was then contemplating the quickest and best way, to get Pat and I to the Sheffield hospital. Again, all manner of things go through your head at such times as these, and I feared that it might be too late to save Rob, by the time the ambulance arrived at the Royal Hallamshire Hospital.

By now, he had been at the Bassetlaw Hospital in excess of an hour, and maybe far too much time had been wasted. If it had not been so chaotic in the A & E department that night, Rob would in my opinion, have been diagnosed much sooner than he was. There was clearly a lack of staff to cope with the flow of incoming patients, most of which, were under the influence of booze, and just required drying out. At the same time, they needed much attention, from the hard-pressed medical team.

At that moment, I spotted Tracey's car approaching across the hospital car park. I made my way to meet her, and informed her regarding the dreadful situation. Fortunately, she had arrived home relatively early that night, and when Pat had broken the news about Rob's accident, without hesitation, Tracey made her way to the Bassetlaw Hospital.

She drove me home, where we had to explain to Pat, how bad things really were. Naturally Pat was now in a state of shock, and disbelief, as she was scurrying around, throwing on some cloths, and tidying her hair. Pat recalls Tracey saying, "Hurry up Mother, you do realise, he could die."

Within a few minutes, we were back in Tracey's car, heading for the Royal Hallamshire Hospital. Tracey can be a fast driver, and she really put her foot down that night. I thought we might catch up with the ambulance, but no, we didn't see any sign of it, and after what seemed like a lifetime, we arrived at the Head Injury Unit. I made enquiries at the reception desk, and we were invited to take a seat in a waiting room. After a few minutes, a nurse came to see us, and she informed us that Rob's condition was critical, and that he had been rushed to theatre, for emergency surgery.

She also said that the surgeon had been unable to wait for our consent to operate, as Rob's situation, was so desperate, to say the least.

It is difficult to describe how you feel in that situation, but I suppose the best words that I can find, are desperate, and frightened. We were then introduced to a senior nursing sister, who would keep us informed as matters progressed. She was very open and honest with us, and gave us some indication of how long the operation might take. It was going to be a very long night, as there was no guarantee that he would survive the operation, and thereafter, it would be some time before we would know the prognosis for Rob's potential recovery. They informed us that usually, someone like Rob, suffering from an intercranial haemorrhage, even if they survive the surgery, there was every chance, that he would be disabled in some way or another. Invasive surgery inside the skull is not good news, and there is always a danger that the patient may not pull through. We were presented with a pamphlet on organ donation, which really focused our minds as to how critical Rob's injury really was. No matter how painful it might be, you have to consider these things, and if Rob was to die, then we should have willingly agreed to any organ donation.

The care from the nursing staff on duty that night was amazing. They showed great empathy, but didn't attempt to underestimate the seriousness of Rob's injury. Cups of tea kept appearing on the scene, and the senior nursing sister looking after our care, put a twenty packet of cigarettes on the table, inviting us to smoke, if we thought it might help. Both Pat and I had stopped smoking several years prior, but without hesitation, we lit one up as we thought it might ease the pain. We were given the privilege of our own visitor's room, which was very considerate, and greatly appreciated. I don't know how many such rooms there are, but for relatives of dangerously ill patients, they certainly are a desirable facility.

Several hours later, the surgeon, Mr P. S. Dais, who had performed the operation came to see us, and he went into great detail, to explain what he had done. Firstly, he apologised for not waiting for our consent, he said that Rob was only minutes away from death, when he arrived in the ambulance. He said that he had removed a blood clot, some three to four inches thick from inside Rob's skull, at the left hand side of his head. He had stopped the bleeding from a severed artery, and now it was just a matter of waiting to see the extent of his internal injuries. He told us that Rob had suffered a haematoma haemorrhage inside his skull. This had been caused by a severe bang to the left hand side of his head, just in front of his ear. Although the brain is cushioned, by the surrounding cerebrospinal fluid in the subarachnoid space, any severe haemorrhage within the relatively rigid skull will ultimately exert pressure on the brain. The degree of pressure, and resultant swelling of the brain, will determine the severity of any brain damage.

The initial prognosis was not good, and it was made perfectly clear that the chances of Rob making a full recovery were very slim. However, with someone of Rob's age, and in such good physical health, there was a reasonable chance, that he could do very well. That said, we were told that the following few days would be critical, and he would be kept sedated, to give his brain the best opportunity to heal. We were informed that he was now on a ventilator, and located in a high dependency facility, receiving intensive care.

That was one of the worst experiences of our life, and it makes you realise how fragile this earthly existence can be. We had retired to bed as usual, not expecting a phone call, giving us bad news like that. I've often heard it said that shocks, and accidents, come along when you are least expecting them. I wondered whether it was the Almighty's way of saying, the Pownall family are having life a little too easy, and I need to slow them down a bit. This probably sounds a crazy notion, but that thought did seriously enter my head.

Although we had the same affection for both our children, it was Tracey that I personally worried about, particularly whenever she was out in her car. This started when she took delivery of her very first car. She had passed her driving test, and some months later she purchased a brand new Fiat Panda. Rob and I went with her to collect the car, and I sat in the front alongside Tracey, with Rob sitting in the rear passenger seat. Her driving was dreadful, and I clearly recall Rob saying that he wished he was wearing his motor cycling crash helmet! I had to insist that she stopped the car, and let me drive it home. When we arrived home, I phoned the guy who had given Tracey her driving lessons, and asked him to provide some further tuition. He came round to collect her, and following a further forty-five minute lesson, he said she was now capable of taking her new car onto the public highway.

At the time, she was working for a bank in Sheffield, and as I was very concerned about her being hurt on the road, I suggested that for a few weeks whist she gained more driving experience, she should take her car to the Worksop train station, leave it there, and then catch the train to Sheffield. She took my advice, and things seemed to be going quite well, as I could see her driving improving, each time she set off up the road.

A couple of weeks later, I was driving on the M1 Motorway en-route to my office in Leeds, when I was overtaken by a bright red Fiat Panda, and I remember thinking that it looked just like Tracey's new car. As I looked more closely, I recognised the number plate, and sure enough, it was Tracey's car. I estimated her speed to be at least 75 mph, as I was cruising along at a steady 65 to 70 mph. I worried all day about this, and when I arrived home, and the four of us were sat down at the dinner table, I said to Tracey, "Did you have a good day at work today," to which she said, "Yes Dad." I then said "Did you leave your car at the train station," and she nodded her head. "You are a lying little devil," I said, "You overtook me on the M1 motorway, travelling at a speed of at least 75 mph." She smiled and said, "Dad, I have been taking my car to Sheffield for weeks now." I trust you can see why I worried about Tracey out on the roads, and never had any real concerns about Rob, as he was a very good driver, having learnt defensive road sense from riding a motorcycle.

I learnt a lot about life that Friday night, not only how you are shocked when something bad catches you unaware, also about life on the streets at night, and some of the things which occur in our hospitals of all places. People like us are cosily tucked up in our beds at night, and we have little concept of the type of things going on within a typical A & E department. There needed to be security people on duty, as the staff were at risk from violence fuelled by drugs, and alcohol. It appeared that the single junior doctor on duty, was under great pressure, and once he realised the serious nature of Rob's injuries, it seemed a long time before he could raise some guidance over the telephone, regarding how to proceed with Rob's urgent situation.

I know it's very difficult, but I do honestly believe that if I had not attended the hospital as I did, then to me, it's likely that Rob would not have survived. I'm not accusing the Bassetlaw medical staff of negligence, but no one knows your family as well as you, and as soon as I set eyes on Rob that night, I knew instinctively that he was in great danger.

I realise that he had been drinking beer, but I don't think for one minute that he was drunk. Pat and I had made a determined effort to educate both our teenage children to appreciate social drinking, without getting bladdered. The stress levels in the Bassetlaw A & E unit that night were unnecessarily high, due to appalling behaviour from patients, under the influence of something, or other. Clearly, the hospital staff were overstretched, and that in itself, creates an environment where things can go wrong. It appeared that the majority of patients including Rob had been drinking alcohol, which says a great deal about the potential dangers from intoxicating drink. Then of course there is the drug situation, and I must admit, that I am very naive about this subject, and wouldn't know how users are likely to react, or be affected whilst under the influence.

Pat and I should like to extend our grateful thanks to the A&E staff at Bassetlaw Hospital, on the night of Friday 12th October 1990, for their efforts in containing Rob's condition, before moving him on for emergency treatment. Although I have made some comments that may be considered controversial; at the end of the day, those looking after Rob that night, did their best under what were difficult, and in my opinion, unfair conditions. We need to look after our medical staff better, particularly those in situations that I have described here. They should not have to work under such pressure, as well as face physical dangers from unruly and abusive patients.

2

High Dependency Care

Having spent Friday night at the Royal Hallamshire Hospital, whilst Rob underwent life saving surgery, we were advised to return to our home and take some much-needed rest. We were mentally, and physically exhausted after what had been a very long and stressful night. A nurse said "make sure you eat something otherwise you won't be in any fit state in a few days time, when we need you to support Rob." It was now a matter of waiting to see how Rob's condition would change following his operation. He was connected to a life support machine with wires and tubes; he lay there looking as though he was in a deep sleep, and it was difficult to accept how poorly he really was.

All three of us visited the hospital later on Saturday, where we were shown to Rob's bed in the high dependency unit. The last thing I wish to do in this chapter is dwell in self-pity. Naturally, like any family faced with this dreadful situation, we were in a state of shock, and very emotional. They had said that it would be a few days before they would have an idea of Rob's likely prognosis. They were looking for a slight improvement each day, but for the first few days following his surgery, there were no real signs of his condition getting better. Brain swelling continued, and this was a major concern, as it was likely to cause damage that would leave Rob with some form of disability. He lay there in just his pyjama trousers, looking remarkably peaceful. Prior to his injury, he had been doing bodybuilding exercises, and this was evident by his muscular upper body. I noticed there were all manner of gadgets placed on a large window ledge behind him; some of them looked like emergency resuscitation devices. There were canister containers with a type of bladder and facemask attached; it all looked very alarming to a non-medical person.

There was a lot of high tech monitoring equipment with flashing LED's (light emitting diodes) and occasionally a buzzer would sound, alerting the attending nurse to something requiring attention. It was the same twenty-four hours a day, as none of the lights on that ward were dimmed during the hours of darkness. Apart from the black sky visible through the large windows, there was no difference in that high dependency unit, between day and night. There was a specialist nurse in full time attendance, with others including doctors, visiting from time to time. This was our very first experience of seeing someone in intensive care, and it was amazing how extensively Rob was being monitored, both from the latest electronic devices, as well as by highly trained staff.

Within the same unit as Rob, there was a little girl who looked about seven or eight years of age. I don't remember her name, but she had been struck by a car, travelling at high-speed, and she had suffered extensive brain damage. It was an incredibly sad sight to see such a beautiful little girl lying there in a coma. She looked perfect, and it was hard to take on board that she was so critically ill. Her bed was covered with colourful cuddly toys, and in an attempt to wake her from the coma; they were playing Jason Donavan records, who was obviously one of her favourite pop stars. There were lots of get-well cards all on display around where she lay. I personally found it very stressful visiting that unit, not only because of Rob's situation, but as soon as I saw that little girl, I couldn't control my emotions. I remember visiting the hospital during those first couple of days, and on one particular occasion at about 03.00am in the morning, when a senior nursing sister explained to me what had happened to this lovely little girl. She said she had been hit by a car, estimated to have been travelling at 60 mph, and her chances of survival were very slim indeed. It was all extremely sad, and I clearly remember her parents coming to visit during those early hours. I shall never forget hearing her mother crying out "Dear God why has this happened to my beautiful child?" Desperation in a person's voice is extremely distressing, and your instincts tell you that you need to do something to help. It made goose bumps appear on my neck, and I felt extremely sick and powerless to do anything about the dire situation.

After a couple of days, we were invited to meet the senior consultant responsible for Rob's care. He outlined the extent of Rob's injuries, and spelt out his chances for a good recovery. Rob's surgery had involved the opening of a section of skull from the left hand side of his head, the removal of a large blood clot, and the sealing of a leakage of blood from the inside of the skull. Rob would be left with an inverted horseshoe shaped scar, some three inches long, and two inches across. The senior consultant emphasised that although medical science had made massive strides in understanding how the human brain works, there is still a lot they don't know. He explained that the will to live is critical to a brain-injured patient, and this is particularly strong in a young person. He addressed me and said, "You and I would now be dead if we had suffered the same injury as Rob. He also referred to the little girl in the next bed to Rob, and explained that although she had suffered severe brain damage, it was always possible that she might wake up at some stage. He said that in some cases, particularly those involving younger patients, parts of the brain virtually unused prior to an injury, could take over from permanently damaged regions. It is thought by the medical profession that in the average person, only ten percent of the total brain capacity is in use at any one time.

It seems that in some cases, the brain has the capability of some kind of re-wiring process, thereby compensating for permanently damaged regions. Why there should be such an excess of functional capacity in the average human brain, is unknown, but maybe it's nature's way of providing options of recovery, when serious head injuries occur.

The senior consultant asked me to be more careful what I was staying at Rob's bedside. He told me it had been observed that I had made comments whilst visiting Rob, and this had caused monitors to sound warnings as he had become increasingly agitated. I can recall saying things that expressed my deep concern for Rob's chances of a good recovery, but I had no idea that he could probably pick up on my murmurings. The consultant explained that although Rob was in a deep coma, it was possible that he could hear every word being said around him. I remember saying "So it's a bit like a brain in a tin can," not a good analogy, but the consultant said, "If you like, yes." This is the stuff horror films are made of, and to me it seemed as if Rob could be experiencing a living hell. The thought of how it might be just lying there, locked in a body, over which you have no control, doesn't really bear thinking about. I remember wondering if Rob was aware of his situation, how he would cope with the passing of time. It wasn't clear whether he might be drifting in and out of consciousness, which would provide some relief, or if he was totally aware of his existence on a continuous basis. It is almost impossible to comprehend what it must be like to experience a coma when you are fully aware, and I could see danger that if it all became too painful to bear, there could be a risk that his brain might go into shut down mode. I was surprised that such patients are not kept in a deeper state of sleep, with absolutely no conscious awareness of what was going on in their world.

Those next few days were very stressful, not knowing whether Rob would survive, and if so, what kind of recovery he would make. We were visiting the hospital twice each day, and this in itself was very tiring. Apart from the travelling time, if we visited in the mid morning, and again in the evening, it all added up to a very long and stressful day. As soon as we arrived home, there was an endless stream of telephone calls from family and friends, all enquiring about Rob's state of health. It's clearly understandable that people wished to show their concern, and find out the latest information, but when you are on the receiving end, it's not easy to show the required level of patience. Pat, Tracey and I were feeling the pressure, not only from the uncertainty of Rob's future, but also from the disruption to our normal daily lives. Sleep was almost non-existent at first, as we were always waiting for the telephone to ring. It was a bit like living on a knife-edge, and it was adrenalin that was keeping us going.

A couple of folks would phone us on a regular basis, and as soon as we answered the call, they would breakdown in floods of tears. It was difficult to know what to say to those people, they were well intentioned, but we didn't really need that kind of contact. By contrast, an ex-manager of mine would call most evenings, give me a good rollicking over too much drink, and not enough food, and that was just what I required. Sympathy was not what I personally needed; positive support was the best option, not some of the daft things that a few well-intentioned folks would say.

My Sister Cynthia, and her husband Cyril, who lived away in Anglesey, were particularly devastated with the news, and Cynthia sent word that she was coming over to Worksop. This was quite understandable, but I contacted one of her sons Kevin, and asked him to politely persuade his mother that now wasn't the time to visit, as we needed our privacy, and would be under even more stress, by additional family staying in the house. Thankfully, she understood, and didn't take any offence. We did our utmost to keep them informed of Rob's situation, as we did with both sides of our family.

It's amazing how people react to this kind of trauma, and I'm sure Cynthia will forgive me for telling how she contacted the Red Arrows for their support.

We were extremely grateful to all our family and friends for their kind thoughts at the time, and although it was stressful, looking back, all those telephone calls were completely understandable.

We found that we needed time; time for just the three of us to reflect on Rob's condition, and feel free to shed a few tears every now and again, within the privacy of our own home. It made me realise how closely linked are the emotions of sadness and humour. I found that following a really good weep; I could almost immediately see the funny side of something, obviously unrelated to Rob's accident.

I have always been a great admirer of the comedian Ken Dodd of Knotty Ash fame. He is a very clever man who plays on the emotions of sadness and humour. He typically sings a very sad song, and whilst you are about to wipe away the odd tear, he then makes you laugh your socks off, just from silly things. I remember Pat and I seeing Ken's act at the Palace Theatre in Manchester. Pat was heavily pregnant at the time with Tracey, and I thought she would give birth. Ken's performance went on long after his allotted time, and we were whipped up into a state of frenzy, laughing at stupid things such as gravy mines, and wading waist high through a bath of custard.

Ken's trick is to make em laugh, and then make em cry; he can do both within a few minutes of each other.

Each member of our family has a strong sense of humour, and I am a very firm believer that this is something you inherit as part of your make up. Rob has always had this wicked humorous side to him, and from a very early age, he would spend a lot of time laughing at things, and situations that amused him. Hopefully, this would assist him in the dark days ahead, and prevent him from slipping into depression.

We did a lot of crying, and I must admit, I felt very guilty, as I was almost continually praying to the Almighty, for him to make Rob better. Whilst I do have some faith in a God of creation, and try very hard to live by a code of conduct set out in the bible, none of our family are regular churchgoers, but we do consider ourselves to be Christians. Pat admits to saying her prayers each evening, and she vowed in prayer to her God, that she would sacrifice anything if Rob could be spared. The experience of Rob's injury did strengthen my faith, and I do genuinely believe that our faith in God gave us strength to cope with the challenges we were facing.

I shall never forget the words written in a get-well card that was sent to our home by Margaret Atack, the wife of a good friend of mine. "The Lord moves in mysterious ways, his wonders to perform."

Back at the hospital, it was now several days since Rob's surgery. He still lay there in a deep coma, connected to the life support machine, with all those tubes and wires. The main problem was that his brain continued to swell, and that created potentially fatal problems from an infarction to the base of his brain. If that was to occur, the result could be complete brain death, or total paralysis from the neck downwards. This was a horrific possibility that was spelt out to us in explicit terms, but all we could do, was to hope and pray that any resultant brain damage would be minimal. They considered easing the pressure by making a large hole in the top of his skull; that would allow his brain to expand, but they decided against it. They kept saying that it was getting time to try to bring him out of his coma. By this time he was on opiate type drugs, and the longer that continued, there would be a potential problem of withdrawal, and addiction. Also, for someone in Rob's situation, the longer they lay there in a comatose state, the less their chances of ever walking again. They suffer from what is known as horse feet, whereby the feet and ankles take on a permanent set in the downward position.

Head injury patients need to be on their feet at the earliest opportunity, even if it is by means of them being supported by a harness; just allowing their feet to be in contact with the ground. It seemed very cruel seeing Rob suspended from a steel cradle, whilst still apparently fast asleep. They made a decision that they would attempt to allow Rob to wake up by slowly reducing his sedation. It was then their intention to take him off the ventilator, providing he could breathe on his own. This failed at the first, and several further attempts, and we now feared that he would never be free of this life support facility. For whatever reason, it seemed to be first thing in the morning when they began bringing him off the breathing machine. Each time they awakened him, he was unable to breathe on his own. He was physically too weak, and became very agitated.

They would inform us when they were taking him off the ventilator, and shortly afterwards, the phone would go again, informing us that he was back on the life support machine. The tensions were indescribable whilst this was taking place, but once they informed us that he was back on the machine, we understood that at least he was more stress free, and hopefully resting peacefully.

We continued with our visits, and whilst Rob's eyes were open, he was totally paralysed, and showed no sign of movement or emotion. I personally hadn't completely given up hope, but I was having very negative thoughts about how things might unfold. It seemed as though there was a different problem each time we visited, but on every occasion, the medical team seemed to have a course of action, and they never wavered in their attempts to restore his state of health. On one visit, we were informed that he had developed pneumonia, and that was a significant set back. You hear of so many seriously ill people dying from pneumonia, and I remember thinking how many more things are there to go wrong.

We visited his bedside, and he looked terrible. His breathing was erratic, and his complexion had taken on a grey colour. I requested another meeting with the senior consultant, and I was determined to push him regarding whether he thought Rob would pull through. I explained our deep anxiety, and said that we would prefer to know the true situation, and then at least, we would be aware of what we were likely to face. Having spelled all this out to the consultant, he looked at me and said, "I think you have given up on Rob, and I'm very unhappy about this. I have a team of highly specialised and dedicated people looking after your son, and despite the ongoing problems including pneumonia, we are still hopeful that he will get better." He explained that pneumonia, whilst being very serious was quite common in a head injury patient such as Rob, and they were treating him with appropriate antibiotics. A senior nursing sister also attended that meeting, and afterwards, she said that she too wished to emphasise the importance of us remaining optimistic about Rob's chances of a good recovery. She suggested that we go home, try to switch off for a little while, and hopefully, Rob would be in a better condition, the next time we visited. That was good for me, and it made me change to a more positive approach, but I was constantly having to battle against those negative thoughts.

The next time we visited Rob, the pneumonia was showing signs of improvement, and this was a considerable boost to our optimism and faith in the treatment Rob was receiving. It's amazing how quickly things can change for someone in that condition. This applies both ways of course, but if the will to live is very strong, it would appear that they are able to keep coming back from the brink, during those early days following a serious head injury.

At one of our evening visit, Pat and Tracey were at Rob's

side, and as usual they were speaking to him, holding his hands, and expressing their deep affection for him; all the time, encouraging him to get better. I was unable to do that kind of thing as I was always overcome by emotion, and I had been given strict orders from the high dependency staff, that it was important to be positive and in control when at Rob's bedside. I would view from a distance, and if it was late at night, I would sit outside the unit in a corridor, generally finding a little discrete corner, and maintain my presence from there. Pat asked Rob to blink an eye if he could understand her, and amazingly he did just that. She tried this again, and it was apparent that he understood her, and for the first time since his injury, he was communicating with her. The medical team looking after Rob were greatly encouraged by this, and for the first time since Rob's injury, we were thinking that he might now make some kind of reasonable recovery. Tracey would sit with him, and following some words of encouragement, she asked him to squeeze her hand if he could understand what she was saying. This worked extremely well, and at least by now, we were able to have some interaction with Rob. Obviously, we had no idea how he was feeling, or what he was thinking about, but at least, if he understood that we were present, and encouraging him, that had to be a good thing.

Looking back, I wish that I could have done more of that kind of thing, which was so important according to the medical team looking after Rob. We all have our strengths and weaknesses, and both Tracey and Pat excelled at Rob's bedside during those dark periods of his coma. My support would be of more value, once I knew that he was going to return to some quality of life.

I remember telephoning the hospital at 08.00am one morning, and they informed me that they had finally managed to get Rob breathing on his own, albeit, supported by oxygen. This was a significant milestone in Rob's recovery, and a considerable boost to our expectations of what might be achieved.

I decided to take a look where Rob's accident had occurred, and located the alleyway, behind what used to be the Gas Showrooms in Watson Road, Worksop. He had needed the toilet urgently, and decided to use this alleyway to spend a quick penny. By now, the alleyway had been fitted with a secure gate, preventing anyone gaining access. Rob had tripped and fallen backwards, dropping approximately five feet into a disused loading chute. Unfortunately, he gave the left hand side of his head a severe crack on the edge of a sharp brick. This was a very dangerous place, and the owner's were obviously concerned about Rob's accident, as they had now made it secure from public access. It's pointless blaming others, but there was an accident waiting to happen with such an unfenced dangerous pit, having open access from the public pavement. I could have forgiven anyone going down that alleyway, as without that recently fitted gate, it wasn't an obvious private right of way.

When you are faced with an almost impossible situation like Rob's accident its easy to blame anyone you can, but both Pat and I agreed to focus on Rob getting better, and praying to the Almighty that he would be spared.

A highly capable surgeon had done his best to repair the damage to Rob's head, and now it was down to Rob himself, as well as the highly trained medical team looking after him, to provide the best possible outcome.

It was now more than one week since Rob's injury, and I had decided to return to my work. I attended a meeting with my manager who had been extremely supportive, and I told him that I needed to get back to my work, as it would prove therapeutic, and although it may sound a little harsh, it would take my mind off Rob's situation, for at least part of the working day. I soon realised that sitting there weeping was not going to solve anything, and I'd be better resuming my occupation, and trying to achieve some kind of normality, at least as far as work was concerned. It wasn't easy for my work colleagues, who found it difficult to know what to say to me. I told them not to feel awkward about the situation, and I would keep them informed regarding Rob's condition. Several of my employer's directors telephoned me on a regular basis, and they were superb. I couldn't have expected any better support during those early troublesome days. Many of my customer contacts were very thoughtful, and showed great concern about Rob's situation. There were a couple in particular who were tremendous, and whilst I'm not naming names, if they do read this book, they will know to whom I'm referring.

I was at my office in Leeds when unexpectedly; the hospital contacted me, and asked if I could attend that afternoon, around 3.00pm. Fearing the worst, I arrived at the high dependency unit, whereupon, I was met by a senior nursing sister. Knowing how emotional I had been, she asked if I could control my emotions sufficiently, to sit down at Rob's side, and explain to him about the cause of his injury. This was not going to be easy for me, but as I was alone with Rob, for some reason, that made the task less stressful. I was shocked when I walked into the high dependency unit to find him out of bed, lying almost upright, in a kind of cradle-cum-chair. There was no expression in his face, just a pitiful staring at the ceiling. Although he was still completely paralysed, they were trying to get some weight onto his feet, at least for a few minutes each day. He looked very uncomfortable slouched in that cradle, but I realised it was in his best interests, to get him out of that bed at every opportunity.

I sat down beside him, and commented that he may not be aware of what had happened, or which hospital was looking after him. Prior to the accident, he had taken delivery of a nice new car, and the thought had crossed my mind that he might be thinking he had been involved in a motoring accident. His new car was his pride and joy, and if he thought it too, had been badly damaged, this would only add to his anxieties. I told him that he had not had a motoring accident; rather, he had had a fall whilst returning home from an evening in town with one of his best mates, Andy Sumpter. There was a nurse looking on and she came up and gave Rob a big hug. She looked at me with a huge smile on her face, and then said, she was delighted, because a single tear had appeared from one of his eyes. I couldn't understand the euphoria, but afterwards she explained that this was the first sign of any emotion, and the next thing would hopefully be a smile.

Looking at Rob again, it all looked very bleak to me, and I couldn't really believe that he was going to have any decent quality of life, ever again. However, the nurse was right, and after a few more days, Rob was showing signs of a faint smile. His mother and sister were saints, and each time they visited, they would chat to him, and all the time, they were encouraging him to get better. A nurse suggested that we take in a photograph of our pet dog Flossy, and they would place it at his bedside, where he could see it, as something like that can be very beneficial in restoring memory etc. Rob thought the world of that dog, and I bet the photograph added to all the encouragement for him to get well again.

Some of Pat's work colleagues bought Rob a present, it was a fury Gorilla. Not what an eighteen-year-old man might expect as a present, but I thought it might bring good fortune, so we decided to sit it on his bedside cabinet. It was a gruesome looking thing with piercing dark brown eyes, but I hoped it would make Rob smile. I spoke to that Gorilla, and asked it to perform a miracle. I still have it, and whilst Pat has often said get rid of it, as it brings back bad memories, it has pride of place in a display cabinet in our garage, and as long as I am alive, that is where it will stay.

Over the following few days, Robs condition gradually improved, although he was still unable to move a limb, or communicate verbally. He had a tracheotomy in his throat, where he was given oxygen, and he was being fed via a tube in his nose. He was still receiving constant supervision by wonderful staff that went to great lengths to make him as comfortable as possible. As he was still unable to blink his eyes subconsciously, periodically, they would apply wipes in order to prevent them becoming dry. Also, as he was unable to clear his throat, at regular intervals, they would insert a suction tube via his tracioctomy, to draw away excess mucus. This made an awful gurgling and squelching sound, but it was something we would have to get used to.

I remember thinking that if I lived to be a very old man, I should never be able to repay my debt of gratitude to our wonderful National Health Service, for the care and treatment of our son Rob.

It seemed very cruel to me, but by now they were getting Rob out of bed, and four physiotherapists were attempting to walk him around the ward. He was unable to support himself, and his body slumped like a limp doll. Two of the lady physiotherapist, were supporting him up on the tips of his toes, whilst the other two were kneeling down behind him, and pushing his legs forward, one at a time. It amazed me how they had the physical strength to hold him up, and manipulate his legs. Again, it looked extremely cruel what they were doing, and it was easy to think that they were fighting a losing battle. These are incredibly capable and determined professional people, who were hopefully going to perform wonders on Rob. There was talk of him having to undergo surgery on the tendons controlling his feet, followed by six months with his lower legs in plaster, to hold his feet in the correct position. Fortunately, this operation was avoided and slowly but surely, they managed to get his feet in a better position, albeit far from where they would need to be, if he would ever walk normally again.

We had to continue combating the negatives, and focus upon the better signs, such as a blinking of the eye, squeezing of the hand, and the occasional smile.

Rob's mates were naturally very upset about his accident, and several expressed a wish to visit him in hospital. For obvious reasons, it was immediate family visiting only, whilst Rob was so dangerously ill, but as soon as he began showing good signs of recovery, we gave our permission for a couple of them to go and see him. Afterwards, we received a telephone call from one of the visitors who described what he had found as, "Rob with tubes and pipes."

We were sitting with a senior nursing sister and reviewing Rob's situation, when she turned to Pat and told her that Rob's best chances of a reasonable recovery, would be for her to give up her employment, and devote herself to looking after Rob fulltime. We had already discussed this ourselves, and had agreed that should he be spared, we would do whatever was required to give him the best quality of life, regardless of commitment or cost. You have to adapt to changing situations in life, and from hereon, our values and life-style would change with new priorities.

We were delighted when they informed us that they were removing Rob from the high dependency unit on to another ward. He was now thankfully out of danger, and it was just a matter of time before we should know what to expect with regards to his physical recovery. The medical team kept reassuring us that the signs were very good, and mentally he was looking extremely strong, and showing every indication that his intelligence and personality, had not been impaired.

By now, Pat and I had given up the cigarettes, and moderated our drinking. After all we thought, its not doing our health any good, and we could well do without the cost. From now on, our lives would be changed, and we had to put all our efforts into ensuring that Rob's needs came first. He was still connected to an oxygen supply by means of his tracheotomy, but this was steadily being reduced, and within a couple of days, he was breathing alone through his nose and mouth. They kept his tracioctomy open in case of an emergency, and then they could re-connect him to the ventilator with great speed. We were visiting one evening when a nurse came to Rob's bedside, and told us that they were going to insert a tube into his tracheotomy. Hopeful, this would enable him to speak a few words. In it went, and the first words we heard were "Hello Mum." This was like a gift from heaven, and things were looking brighter all the time.

They allowed me to cut Rob's hair very short, because as it was, it looked ridiculous, with the part round his wound shaven, and the remainder of it rather long. I took my haircutting scissors to the hospital, and gave him a short back and sides. I had to avoid the dressing, and stay well clear of the wound, but he now looked more like our handsome son had appeared prior to his accident.

A work colleague of mine, and a good family friend, expressed a wish to see Rob in hospital, and arrangements were made for an afternoon visit. I remember him making Rob smile when he suggested that Rob should try smoking a cigarette through the hole in his tracheotomy tube. He was miming the suggestion by holding an imaginary cigarette to his throat, and it really was amusing. Rob needed a good laugh, and this visit did him a lot of good.

During one evening visit, Tracey Pat and I were at Rob's bedside, when Rob suddenly coughed, and out shot his tracheoctomy tube, skidding across the floor. I admit that I panicked, thinking that Rob might choke or suffocate in seconds. I ran to the nurse's station, and asked them to attend to him immediately. When the nurse saw what had happened, she gave me a big smile, washed the tube, and gently replaced it.

I clearly remember during one visit being advised by a senior member of staff to sue the Bassettlaw District Hospital for neglect. She said there had been some considerable delay in diagnosing Rob's serious condition, and if they had referred him to the Royal Hallamshire Hospital much sooner, he would no doubt be looking at a complete recovery. Neither Pat nor I would have anything to do with that and although maybe we would have had a case, and it was likely that he might have been awarded a large amount of compensation, it was not what we wanted to do. I had been at the Bassetlaw District Hospital and seen first hand the enormous pressure both the doctor and nurses on duty were under that night, and I personally thought if we do something like that, the Lord would avenge us in another way. Those on duty at the Worksop A & E department had done their best under very difficult circumstances. We were just grateful that Rob was still alive, and by now it was looking increasingly likely that his recovery would be better than we had first feared. There's no validity in trying to pinpoint blame, Rob was unlucky enough to have a serious accident that could have happened to anyone. He should not have gone down that alleyway, but knowing what it's like when you've had a few beers and you require the toilet, needs must and you take whatever action to seek appropriate relief. From now on, it was going to be down to Rob's courage and determination that would influence the extent of his progress.

The majority of other patients on Rob's new ward were being treated for brain tumours, and I distinctly remember a guy in the bed opposite. I do not recall his name but Rob struggled to explain how kind this chap had been towards him, and how he had kept reassuring Rob that he would be okay. Rob commented that this guy was terminally ill, and had only a few days to live. Rob asked if I would go and sit with the guy, as he had not received any visitors since Rob had been on that ward. I went over and thanked the man for being so kind towards Rob. I asked him if he was expecting any visitors, and he informed that he had no surviving family, and very few friends. He told me that although he had received surgery, there was nothing that could be done as he had a cancer that completely encircled his brain, and it was untreatable. He said the medical team had been very open with him, and told him that he had only about ten days to live. I asked him if I could get him anything, and suggested that he might wish to partake in a few beers. He said he would very much appreciate some beers, so I made my way to the nurse's station, and asked their permission, before making my way to a nearby off-licence. I found myself extremely inadequate in that situation, and it was difficult to know what to say to him. It's amazing how courageous some individuals can be when faced with the onset of premature death. He was amazingly cheerful and grateful when I returned with the beers. He asked if I minded him sharing the beers with some other guys on the ward, and of course that wasn't a problem for me. He said they would wait until after visiting time, before cracking the beer cans open. It was nice to be able to bring just a little pleasure to such a brave man who had so generously supported Rob. I could almost imagine someone with only a few days to live, having resentment for a younger guy, with a great deal of his life still ahead of him.

We didn't see that chap again, because the following day, Rob was relocated to the Lodge Moor Hospital in Sheffield, where ongoing treatment would be provided. At the time of Rob's transfer from The Royal Hallamshire to Lodge Moor, he could sit up unaided but was unable to walk. By now he was taking very light foods by mouth, but he could not handle a knife and fork. The physiotherapists had worked very hard trying to stretch the tendons in the back of Rob's legs, and slowly, his feet were improving, but they still had a long way to go before they would return to a more normal position. We were told that he would be required to stay at Lodge Moor for a period of at least two months, but that was not a problem, as long as we could see a continual improvement.

Lodge Moor would be a further distance to travel, and maybe we would have to consider cutting down on the frequency of our visits. It would all depend on Rob's progress, and how he was shaping up psychologically, to a long spell in hospital. The only other time he had been in hospital prior to his injury was when he was about 7 or 8 years of age. We were living in Leicester at the time, and Rob was admitted to the Leicester Royal Infirmary to have his tonsils removed. We took him in one afternoon, and he had the operation the following morning. They advised us to visit him about four o'clock that afternoon, and when we arrived, he looked in an awful state. There was a lot of blood on his pillow, and sheets, and he was swearing in a manner that was more than a little embarrassing! Fortunately, he was much better the following day, and it was a relief to get him back home.

We shall always be indebted to the staff at the Royal Hallamshire Hospital for their services in saving Rob's life. The quality of care was amazing and there wasn't one single member of staff that didn't show feeling, and empathy, when we were most in need of their support. Whilst all the staff were professional, and kind, in particular, I should like to extend our sincere and grateful thanks to the senior consultant in charge of Rob's care, the very clever surgeon, Senior Registrar in Neurosurgery, Mr Palitha S. Dias FRCS (England) FRCS (Surg Neurol), who did his bit by putting Robs head back together again, and all other doctors and nurses who did such a splendid job by saving our son's life. If it hadn't been for the immediate action by Mr Dias, when

Rob arrived that dreadful Friday night, it's doubtful whether he would have survived. We owe such a great deal to people like these who have dedicated themselves to healing the sick. On the other hand, they must get immense satisfaction when they are able to bring someone, particularly a young person, back from the brink.

If I could change anything during those critical days it would be my negativity about Rob's prospects. I suppose it was the shock of seeing your son in a comatose situation that makes you think that he might not survive. There was always the possibility that he would not come through the darkness that had embraced him, but I should have had more faith in those looking after him, and had greater trust in the Almighty. At the end of the day, you are what you are, and I suppose I was, how I was, because I found it too painful to bear the loss of a teenage son, and feared the prospects of Rob having a future with no real quality of life. Having now seen several miracles happen in the course of the past few weeks, I was going to be in a better state of mind to support him during his long road through rehabilitation.

The monetary cost of Rob's surgery, and treatment at the Royal Hallamshire Hospital, must have been enormous. Unfortunately, he was just one of a steady stream of similar patients requiring this highly expensive care. Maybe, we shall find a way of paying something back, once Rob finally returns home.

The only criticism I have towards The Royal Hallamshire Hospital is one that I guess applies to most hospitals in this day and age, and that is the lack of car parking spaces. Also the cost, as when you are visiting a patient several times per day, over a long period of time, the cost is considerable. I would propose that hospitals should consider multi-storey car parks, when available land is at a premium. I know that planning permission might be difficult due to their unsightly nature, but surely, those visiting loved ones, and in a state of anxiety, should be able to park their vehicles with relative ease, and at minimal or no cost to them. When faced as we were, with Rob's situation, you are under enough pressure when visiting, without the hassle of driving round, sometimes for ages, searching of a place to park your car. This in no way diminishes our appreciation of what the hospital did for Rob, and we are just grateful that such places are available when you most need them.

Thanks again to all the staff at the Royal Hallamshire Hospital (Head Injury Unit); we shall always remember your excellent work.

3

Rehabilitation

Rob was moved from the Royal Hallamshire Hospital in the centre of Sheffield, to Lodge Moor Hospital, which is located on the northern outskirts of the city. At first it looked a fairly run down place, but we very soon discovered that it was an excellent environment for Rob to continue his recuperation. At the time of his admission, he was unable to walk, and could not even hold a knife and fork, let alone use them. His speech was slowly returning, but required a lot of work to improve the strength, and quality of the sounds, and pronunciation. He was dependant upon a wheelchair for getting around, and needed someone to push him along. He could now support his head in an upright position, and was able to sit up on his own, but that was about the extent on his bodily mobility.

It was becoming very evident that any brain damage had not impaired his intelligence or personality. His problems appeared to be purely physical, but I'm sure there were physiological scars, perfectly understandable in an 18-year-old man, who had lost the physical use of his body, and would no doubt be wondering whether he would ever walk again.

The strain at home was beginning to show, and we had to work hard to keep our relationship intact. Although we were pre-warned about the statistics of break-ups following events such as Rob's injury, it was now becoming a reality. We were determined that we would not fall victim to this happening to us, and thankfully, we worked our way through the bad times. Looking back it wasn't such a big deal, the relationship was sound, and it was purely the stress of not knowing what we would have to face that brought tension to the fore.

It was good to see Rob in different surrounds away from the critically ill environment of the Royal Hallamshire Hospital wards. He now needed some stimulation to get him up on his feet, and moving around. His body looked very weak, and a far cry from his physical fitness prior to his head injury. Goodness knows what he would have been like at this stage, had he not been in great condition prior to his accident.

I guess it's easy for someone in Rob's situation to settle for an easy life, and not commit to the strenuous regimes that were set before him. After all, there are many similar individuals that don't have a choice, and have to resign themselves to being confined to a wheelchair. Rob was having none of this, and his determination strengthened the belief that he would one day walk out through those hospital doors. I was concerned that he was driving himself too hard, and that if progress became too difficult to achieve, or even impossible, he might sink into depression. There was no shortage of encouragement, both from the medical staff, as well as from fellow patients, and thankfully my fears about Rob's progress, were ill founded.

As a family, Tracey, Pat and I were obviously able to contribute to his motivation, through encouragement and support. Both the staff and other patients were all very pleasant people, and Rob seemed to settle in nicely, for what was going to be a rather long stay. I wondered how he would resign himself to several months in hospital, but I needn't have been concerned, because he never became unsettled, or complained about the loss of his freedom.

Initially, he was put on a large open ward with his bed situated in the top right hand corner, from the entrance doors. To begin with, he was in a bed with sides to prevent him falling onto the floor. Very soon, the sides of the bed were lowered during the day, and then raised at night-time. What we didn't realise at first, was that Lodge Moor was a multi purpose hospital, and in addition to patients such as Rob requiring long-term recovery from very serious injuries, it also served as a respite hospital, as well as a hospice.

There were all kinds of potential hurdles ahead, but very slowly, progress was being made. He recalls being hoisted into the bath, and one day when he was wheeled into the bathroom, there stood a pretty student nurse. He was asked whether she could attend, whilst he was bathed as part of her training. Rob declined saying "Please give me bit of dignity." He wouldn't have intended any offence, but it is understandable that he would not wish an attractive young lady, looking on at his frail and distorted body.

Rob's first salutary lesson was, you should always remember to apply the brake to the wheelchair, whenever it was stationary. He describes a situation early on, where he had not activated the brake, and as he leaned forward to place something down on his bed, the chair shot back, and he found himself on all fours, on the ward floor, with his backside in the air, and unable to move from that position.

I stated earlier that all the time Rob was recovering from his injury, we had never found him depressed or unhappy. He does however, admit that one day, not long after being admitted to Lodge Moor Hospital, he was feeling a bit low, and a male nurse came to him and asked what was the matter. Rob said "Wouldn't you be pissed off if you were in my situation." Rob said the nurse left him alone, which probably seems quite harsh, but in Rob's words, "It was the best thing he could have done, as he was treating me like an adult."

Rob describes treatment at Lodge Moor on day one as horrible. He says he was wheeled into a physiotherapy room, where he was sat on a bench in front of a large mirror. He says he couldn't recognise what was staring back, and best describes it like a skinny, but pot bellied, pale, tired looking man, sat in the most contorted, and twisted way, the body is able to achieve. A lot of Rob's treatment was about straightening him out, his ankles being one of the biggest problems.

There was a real mixture of patients on the ward, and I suppose that was a good thing, as they could support each other, a bit like a large family unit. There were a number of elderly gentlemen approaching the end of their days, and this of course was very sad. One old gentleman that I particularly remember was a nice little chap by the name of Frank. I believe he was suffering from dementia, and was probably in Lodge Moor to give his wife a break from the responsibility of looking after him. Frank was generally fully dressed during the daytime, and he would shuffle around the ward, talking to anyone who would engage in conversation. He was able to recall many things from World War 2, and beyond, but he wouldn't have a clue as to what had happened an hour ago. He was also known to get out of bed at night, and wander around the ward. One night Rob had a shock in the middle of the night, when he awoke to discover that Frank was trying to get in bed with him. Frank's bed was in a little side ward, and Rob remembers just prior to Christmas when the main ward had been decked with decorations, Pat and I were visiting, and poor old Frank had a panic attack, thinking that the glistening decorations were on fire. He remembers me visiting Frank in his side ward, attempting to calm him down.

Another elderly gentleman with Alzheimer's disease, would occasionally parade around the ward naked, during the course of the night. An ex-holiday representative was receiving rehabilitation therapy, following a cerebral bleed.

He was struggling psychologically to come to terms with his disabilities, and the staff were working very hard to keep him feeling positive, and motivated about his rehabilitation. There was another elderly gentleman named George, who was confined to a wheel chair. He and Rob became very goods friends, and although we didn't realise it at the time, George was terminally ill, and the end was quite near.

At the opposite end of the ward was a young man of similar age to Rob, who lay in a coma. He had been in that state for a period of eighteen months, following a serious motoring accident. We noticed that he didn't have many visitors, and I guess that was understandable, after such a long time in a coma. You have to wonder how relatives cope with a situation like that, and after such a long time without any communication, I suppose there seems little point in visiting on a daily basis.

Another patient was an ex-coal-miner, who was suffering from a fused spinal injury. He was unable to sit down, and at meal times he would stand at the communal table, and eat from an extended tray. Rob recall's someone saying to the chap "Take a seat mate, don't just stand there." This seams like bad humour, but as Rob says "When you're all in a bad way, anything goes and nobody took offence.

Rob has very fond memories of a particular nursing sister on the ward, also an older nurse, who referred to the patients as her boys. I can see her now strutting into ward, and in a loud voice saying, "How are you my boys?" She was very much a motherly figure, who showed great care for all her patients. She would occasionally confide in Pat and I, by telling us off the record, that she believed Rob's eventual outcome would be very good.

Visiting Rob at Lodge Moor was very time consuming, but we felt the necessity to see him each day, although some weekdays, it was just me as I was en route home from my office in Leeds. There was an off-licence close to the hospital, and most nights, I would stop and buy Rob a pint bottle of Guinness. Knowing that he enjoyed a drink, I thought the stout would help build him up, following his injury.

They were very long days, but we got on with it, as we wanted to give Rob every encouragement in his quest to regain his mobility.

At first, it seemed that Rob had a real up hill battle in front of him, but we could detect from the start that he had determination, and was prepared to give it his best shot. The first thing they focused upon was to teach him to hold a knife and fork. Initially, this took place whilst he was propped up in his bed, and it was very painful to see the extent of his disability. We take these and many other skills for granted having leant them during our childhood. Having to learn how to do something as basic as using your cutlery as an adult, seemed very difficult indeed.

I remember quite early on with this training, Pat and I arrived just as a cooked lunch was being served. We sat at Rob's bedside, and he was just how an infant would be in trying to pick up the knife and fork. Pat took pity on him, and began feeding him as you would with a small child. A nurse appeared on the scene, and when she witnessed what was happening, she very abruptly instructed Pat to stop helping him immediately. She insisted that he had to learn for himself, and whilst it might seem cruel, it was the only way for him to acquire this basic skill. It struck me that the old saying 'There's no gain without pain' is particularly poignant, when you are involved in rehabilitation. We had to be as tough as Rob, and allow him to soldier on, and not feel sorry for him.

Lodge Moor operated a strict and tough regime, for rehabilitation patients such as Rob. Each day began at 7-30am, and there was never an opportunity of a lie in. After breakfast, Rob and others requiring therapy, were wheeled down to the appropriate area, and work began until lunchtime. They would break for lunch, and then it was work again in the afternoon. At the end of the day, Rob was really tired, and usually when we visited in the evening, we would find him relaxing in his bed.

As well as physical exercises, Rob received intensive speech therapy, not only to develop his vocal capabilities, but also to determine whether or not he had suffered a dysphagia from his accident. Disphagia following a serious head injury can cause problems with swallowing, which obviously would mean ongoing problems regarding dietary matters.

Swallowing is a complex process requiring many nerves, and muscles for it to operate properly. Part of the act of swallowing is under voluntary control, which means you are aware of controlling the action. However, much of the swallowing process is involuntary. Robs injuries had left him with problems in his soft pallet that impeded his speech. However, they found that he was not affected by dysphagia. Robs speech therapy involved making sounds such as 'mmmmm', 'ba', 'mmmmm', 'ba', which were intended to strengthen the soft pallet, by switching the sound from his mouth, to his nasal passages, and vice versa.

As soon as he was able to move himself around in his wheel chair, he had to attend the communal table, where all patients that were physically able, would eat all their meals. I could see the logic behind this, as it provided some social interaction with fellow patients, and I suppose in Rob's case, it gave some peer pressure to improve his handling of the cutlery. Everyone around that table had some problems to cope with, and there seemed to be a good camaraderie between young and old alike.

Over the next few weeks, the staff worked wonders on Rob, and following an abundance of determination on his part, slowly, but surely, they were helping him regain the use of his limbs. They kept me busy massaging his calf muscles, which was intended to stretch the tendons in the back of his legs. It was quite hard work, and Rob would complain that I was pulling out the hairs in his legs. We had to complete this massage every day, as it was essential that those tendons become extended, before he could attempt to walk again.

Rob's injury had certainly not changed his sense of humour, and most evenings when I visited him, he would have something amusing to relate. Very often at the weekend, when both Pat and I would be visiting him in the evening, we would leave him in fits of laughter. It was remarkable how his spirits kept up, and there was never an occasion when we found him depressed. I could have understood if he despaired at the very long road ahead. This was the time of his life, when he should be having fun, and enjoying himself, not stuck in a hospital having to push himself to the limit, each and every single day. He just kept pushing, and pushing and slowly, we could see that he was making steady progress.

In the early days, they worked on him gaining strength in his upper body and arms. They would sit him down on a bench, and the ask him to sit up straight. When he thought he was holding a good posture, they would put a mirror in front of him, and he would be shocked at how he appeared. The problem stemmed from contorted back muscles that needed to be relaxed. He also required the strength in his upper arms to increase, so that he would be able to support himself in, and out of his wheel chair. When they started to get him up on his feet, they physically supported him from either side, and encouraged him to move his legs. It was a number of weeks before they got him to balance on his feet, and I can clearly remember the excitement all-round when eventually he made his very first step. Rob clearly remembers when this happened, he says, "Admittedly, I was holding onto a bar, but at least I had managed my very first step."

Following a period where the two physiotherapists were supporting him, one on either side, and when he had gained more strength in his arms, they had him trying to walk between two handrails, and at first it looked as though he had wooden legs. It was very hard work, and in the evenings you could see that he was tired, and in need of much rest. Never did they suggest, or encourage, the use of a walking frame or a stick, as they believed he might become dependant upon such a device, and as painful as it may seem, they forcefully encouraged him to walk unassisted.

A couple of weeks later and Rob managed to walk back into the ward. Very, very slowly, he put one foot in front of the other, and the ward staff gathered to watch. They were all clapping their hands in appreciation of his hard work, and Rob describes that moment as one in which he felt very proud indeed. He had worked extremely hard for this to happen, and although it was only a few steps, it represented another significant milestone. He made a pledge that he would not leave the hospital unless he could walk out unaided, and at the time when he made that commitment, I must admit that I thought he was being very optimistic.

We found it remarkable that Rob's attitude remained so positive about the future, and his sense of humour never faltered, at least not in our eyes. He was eating enormous amounts of food, and the very first time I saw his evening meal, I couldn't believe my eyes. It was ridiculous, so much so, that I queried it with a nurse. She explained that this was perfectly normal for someone like Rob, recovering from a serious head injury, and he would consume such amounts of food for up to six months after his injury. The food was of excellent quality, intended to provide an abundance of nutrition, for those like Rob, involved in daily, physically demanding exercises. We were also informed that brain damaged patients need vast amounts of nourishing food to heal their wounds.

Time slowly passed by, and we were given instructions on how to assist Rob in and out of a wheel chair. It's all about balance, and as Rob was quite a big fellow, I had to be careful that we both didn't lose balance, and finish up in a heap on the floor. We soon got used to it, and we passed the test, so that we would soon be allowed to take him outdoors. Rob had to sit on the side of the bed, and then we would assist him to stand on his feet, whilst I stood facing him. Then, with his wheelchair close by, it was a matter of swinging him round, and lowering him into his chair. We were also asked to think about him coming home, initially for one night, just to see how we could all manage. We would need to have a bed downstairs, as climbing stairs would be out of the question, for a very long time. I remember making a ramp, so that we could access the back door, when it was time for Rob to come home in his wheel chair. Eventually, the wonderful day arrived, and we were advised that initially Rob should come home, for one Friday evening. It was all very emotional, but we kept ourselves together, and all the family was very excited. It was a bit of a struggle assisting Rob into the car from his wheelchair, but we managed it, and we were soon on our way to Worksop.

This was a day that sometimes, I never thought would happen. It was just an overnight stay, but we were going to make the most of it. Shortly after our arrival home, Rob expressed some concern about having the bed down stairs, although he had been made well aware of the situation, whilst discussions about his venture home had taken place. It was apparent that he was not happy about having a bed downstairs, but he had to get on with it. I suppose having the bed downstairs was generally associated with an elderly and infirm person, approaching the end of their days. His first visit home passed by all too quickly, and after tea on Saturday afternoon, we had to take him back to Lodge Moor.

The following Friday arrived, and Rob was coming home for the second time. When we arrived home, he looked at me and said, "I bet between us, we could get me upstairs." He said there was nothing he would wish for more than to have a night in his own bed, in the privacy of his bedroom. His mother was dead against the idea, but I thought it might be worth a try. Pat was concerned that we should be in big trouble if anything went wrong, and we had to call for assistance. She was worried that we might undo the remarkable progress already made, if he was to take another fall.

We enjoyed our evening together, and then it was time for bed. I wheeled Rob to the bottom of the stairs, and then assisted him to stand up and park his backside on the bottom stair. The plan was for him to go up backwards, in a sitting position, taking one step at a time. It was a real struggle, but between us we made it to the top, and Rob had a good night sleep, in his very own bed. Having managed to get him up stairs, I was then worried about getting him down again the following morning. I needed to be concerned, because arguably it was more difficult, with potentially increased danger that he might fall on top of me, and we could both have come crashing down. Taking our time, we made it, and agreed that for all future home visits, we would endeavour to get Rob up the stairs, and into his own bed. I told him not to say a word to anyone at the hospital, about our cunning deed, as it might get me into trouble.

Following a couple of successful, single overnight home visits, Rob was allowed to stay from Friday evening until

Sunday night. It was great picking him up on a Friday on my way home from Leeds, but Pat and I found it very sad having the take him back after Sunday night's tea.

Christmas was fast approaching and Rob had set himself a target of walking out of the hospital unaided. I personally thought he was being overly ambitious, but he did it. It was rather tense as there was snow on the ground, and the last thing he needed was another fall. I parked the car as close to the hospital door as possible, and he walked out very slowly, a bit like a tin soldier.

Rob had requested an electric guitar as a Christmas present, and it had to be a red one. He explained that playing this instrument would improve the dexterity in his hands and fingers, as well as being another interest. We were able to meet his request, and all the preparations for a wonderful Christmas had been completed. The shiny red guitar was already wrapped, and all the customary goodies were organised.

The weather was really bad over that Christmas period, and a substantial snowfall had brought down electricity lines, resulting in power cuts, for a couple of days over the holiday. Fortunately, I had a Calor gas camping stove, that we used for cooking and we all huddled around the gas fire to keep ourselves warm. Rob sat with a sleeping bag wrapped around him, looking a bit like 'Nanook of the North!'

Christmas day was fine, with no electricity cuts; therefore, we were able to cook the Christmas dinner with all the customary trimmings. Guitar practice was underway, but I doubted whether Rob would ever become the next Bert Weedon or Eric Clapton. That didn't matter a jot, and it was just good to see him achieving these goals.

As part of Rob's ongoing assessment, it had been decided that providing we managed all right over the Christmas holidays, he should return to Lodge Moor Hospital for one more week's intensive physiotherapy, and then he would be discharged. By this time, Rob could walk unaided for a minimal distance but it obviously required tremendous physical effort, and the technique had a great deal to be desired. We were very impressed, and pleased with the good work put into Rob by the staff at Lodge Moor Hospital. I don't recall ever finding him depressed throughout his two-month stay, which I find remarkable considering the extent of his disability. On the contrary, we very often left Rob in hysterics, after giving us some amusing stories about events on the ward. It was apparent that Rob was very popular with all the nurses and patients alike. As I have stated earlier, one nurse in particular would often say to us that in her opinion, Rob would make an excellent recovery. She was right of course, but it didn't come easy, and although we were very pleased about his progress whilst staying at Lodge Moor Hospital, he still had a very long way to go, in order to improve his mobility. Following a wonderful Christmas holiday, Rob returned to Lodge Moor for one final week.

Prior to Christmas, Rob had asked his friend George if he would be going home for the holiday. George responded by saying he had decided to stay in hospital, as he wished to be remembered as the guy sat at the head of the table, carving the turkey, and not someone in a wheel chair. Sadly, when Rob returned to Lodge Moor Hospital after Christmas, George had passed away. This was another blow to Rob, which he coped with admirably.

I collected him on the Friday evening on my way home from work, and as before at the time of the Christmas holiday, he insisted upon walking out of the hospital unaided. It was a bit emotional, and it reminded me of that scene from the Dam Busters film, where Douglas Bader took his first steps on his artificial legs. I think Rob found it a bit tough saying good-bye to the nurses and fellow patients.

After all, he had got to know some of them extremely well, and no doubt he would miss them for some considerable time.

From now on, life would be very different, and of course all the visiting would be over. Pat gave up her job as manageress of Thurston's bread and confectionery shop, so that she would be available full time, to support Rob from there on. Lodge Moor Hospital is now closed, and the site has been converted into a housing development. The Pownall family including Rob have a debt of gratitude to Lodge Moor that we shall never forget.

Rob recalls a doctor visiting our home sometime after he had been discharged from Lodge Moor Hospital. The purpose of this visit was to assess Rob's progress, and check for certain ongoing problems. After the physical checks, the doctor turned to me and asked whether I had detected any mood changes in Rob, following his accident. He asked if he had become more aggressive and I said, "No he's always been like that." The doctor looked somewhat alarmed, but I explained that my remark was only intended as a joke, and he could be assured that we had not sensed any mood, or behavioural changes, whatsoever.

Having been discharged from Lodge Moor Hospital, Rob was now required to attend a Head Injury Rehabilitation Unit in Sheffield. This was to take place early in the new year of 1991, and continue until May the same year. It was only one half day each week, but that was enough for Rob, as he didn't like the place, mainly due to the attitude of some members of the staff. He never complained about any of the staff at the Hallamshire Royal Infirmary or Lodge Moor Hospital, but right from the beginning, he was not happy at the Head Injury Rehabilitation Unit, mainly because of one lady in particular. He came home annoyed that she had given him exercises to do, that he found totally impossible. I suspected that they purposely set very ambitious goals, in the belief that rehab has to be hard, and there's no place for pussy footing around, when you have mountains to climb. Having said that, I do suspect there were a few personality issues with certain members of staff, because Rob is a very easy guy to get on with, and his determination to achieve a high standard of recovery, was never in question. He never once complained about the physiotherapists at either of the previous hospitals even when challenged, with the most physically demanding exercise routines.

As it was going to be difficult for me to transport Rob to and from the Rehab Unit, we were offered the services of one of those voluntary taxis. It's a very good cause, and those who volunteer their time to transport people to and from hospital, using their own vehicles, are to be commended, and admired. However, on the very first visit, would you believe it, the taxi was involved in an accident en route to Sheffield? I was at my office in Leeds, when I received a call from the Rotherham General Hospital, asking me to attend as soon as possible. I couldn't believe this, and as I drove to Rotherham from Leeds, I was wondering how I should find Rob, following yet another accident. I didn't know how his head would stand up to another bang, and had there been enough time for it to fully heal? I walked into the A & E department, not knowing what I would find, and there he lay on a trolley, not looking anywhere near as bad as he was when I first saw him, following his major accident. It wasn't as bad as it might have been, although in the accident, Rob had taken another knock to his previously damaged head. Following an x-ray, and some tests, he was allowed to return home, and then of course, we had to break the news to his mother, who naturally, couldn't believe what had occurred.

Afterwards, Rob described what had happened, and he said he could see the accident coming, as the driver was getting on a bit, and not fully in control of the vehicle. It's a magnificent service that many retired individuals provide, but following Rob's experience, I do wonder whether it's such a good idea, and that whilst some volunteers have the best of intentions, there ought to be better screening of those taking part. For me, that was the end of the voluntary taxi service, and from then on, I had to find time in my busy working schedule, to transport him for his once a week, rehabilitation session.

As I have stated earlier, my employer, James Walker & Co Ltd, was extremely considerate following Rob's accident. They offered me the very best support, for which Pat and I shall always be grateful. A few weeks after Rob had been discharged from Lodge Moor Hospital, I received a telephone call from the national sales manager, to say he had noticed that my company car was due for renewal. He said the company wished to help us in anyway they could, but they were limited in what they could do. He pointed out that my company car allocation, did not cover the additional cost of an estate model, but he had observed someone struggling to get a wheelchair into the boot of a saloon car, and if I wished, the company would allow me to have an estate car. We were very grateful, and took up this kind offer. It proved to be a blessing, as we would require the use of a wheel chair, for many months to come.

Rob's physical disability problems resulted from brain damage, restricting certain signals to parts of his anatomy, which all serve to facilitate the process of mobility, and walking. He was left with numerous physical problems, including stiffness in his back and legs, weak ankles, and increased sensitivity, to the soles of his feet. Walking was never going to be easy for Rob, and even after all the physiotherapy that he had whilst at Lodge Moor Hospital, the Rehab Unit were effectively going to teach Rob to walk, the best he could, accepting that from now on, he would always experience, substantial difficulties. The first thing they did was to explain the normal walking process, which in itself is quite complex. It's amazing how we humans walk around, without any real conscious thought. It's something that we take for granted, but the mechanics involved, are really very complicated. Many muscles are involved, and to be able to walk normally, the large muscles at either side of the lower back, have to tense and relax alternatively, from side to side. In reality, for normal walking, you effectively fall forwards with one leg, and then recover through your balance.

Rob's injury left him with brain damage that caused him to have impaired neurological signals, from the brain, to three quarters of the way down his back, as well as to his feet. Having gone to great lengths to explain the normal walking process, the physiotherapists at the Sheffield Rehab Unit, started training Rob to walk as well as possible, taking into account his disability.

No longer would walking be a subconscious process, and for the remainder of his life, he will have to consciously think about what he is doing. Both sides of the muscles in Rob's lower back, no longer release automatically, as they do in natural walking, therefore, he has to balance and physically force each leg forward, one at a time. The visual effect of his new style of walking appears robotic, and the Rehab nurses provided lots of help, with concealing this tin soldier effect to a minimum. They had him walking towards a mirror, so that he could see for himself how his walking appeared to others. He was also videoed, again, so that he could view his walking from other angles. This was all good stuff, and the improvements were very evident.

Whilst Rob did not particularly get on with the staff at the Rehab Unit, certainly nowhere near as much as he did with the Royal Hallamshire and Lodge Moor Hospital staff, in my opinion, they did a good job, in improving his style of walking.

One great difficulty for Rob is climbing, and worse still, descending stairs; this is because the tendons in his legs were shortened due to lying in a coma for about ten days. He suffers from a heightened reaction from his feet, to sensitivity. If someone tickles adult's feet, the automatic reaction is to repel, whereas, in an infant, the tendency is to push down. That's why; Rob now refers to him having an infantile reaction, from the sensitivity in his feet. It is very difficult for Rob to climb down stairs, because his feet are automatically forced forward, which has a similar effect to walking down stairs, on your tiptoes.

Something that Rob had to work very hard at was to avoid becoming self-conscious when walking into a room full of people. Following a serious head injury, it's not only the physical scars that remain, but there are psychological difficulties to be overcome and cope with. Anyone can feel a little self-conscious walking into a room full of people, but for the likes of Rob, this experience is far more significant.

We are grateful to the staff of the Sheffield Rehab Unit, for their professional training, plus detailed education on the walking process, and how Rob should best handle his walking disability, into the future.

Rob remembers a number of fellow attendees to the Head Injury Unit, including a guy who had suffered a serious head injury in a motoring accident, plus another car crash patient, who was struggling to come to terms with the fact that all his passengers in the car at the time of his accident had been killed. There was another dreadful case of a young man who had been hit on the back of his head by a baseball bat, whilst he had been standing at an arcade pinball machine. The back of his skull had been smashed to pieces, and they were still debating whether or not to fit a steel plate, as part of his ongoing treatment.

I am ashamed to say that one day when Rob and I were visiting the Rehab Unit; we were struck with the giggles, when we saw the behaviour of some severely disabled individuals. It doesn't take much to start Rob off laughing, as from a small boy he has always had a very strong sense of humour, sometimes out of control, and this could cause some embarrassment. It's a dreadful situation to be in, when you are unable to avoid laughing at a person's disability. You feel shame and a lack of self-control, and you become greatly embarrassed when all you can do is laugh. I suppose it is a human failing to laugh at someone's misfortune, or disability.

I remember the time Pat, Rob and I, were at Manchester airport, when we were going on one of those post accident holidays. Rob had gone to the bar for some drinks, and as he walked across the airport lounge, we could see people staring at him, and passing comment. As he stood at the bar, a very badly disabled person, far more disabled than Rob, came walking past, and not a single individual took any notice. It appeared that this young man had suffered from something like rickets, as his legs were very badly deformed. It was pitiful to watch the poor guy struggling along on his twisted limbs, but not one person in the surrounding area, paid any attention whatsoever. We then spotted Rob returning with his drinks, and again, we could see people laughing at him. Pat was very annoyed, and said she wanted to give someone a slap. I was more understanding, and I could see that they might have thought he was drunk, as sometimes his stiff walking was similar to how someone under the influence of drink, might appear.

We never saw anyone laughing at Rob's walking after that, which was a blessing, and probably, because he worked very hard at improving the style. Walking can be very amusing, and some of you reading this book might remember the comedian Max Wall, with his hilarious comedy walk, or more recently, John Cleese, in that classic comedy sketch, when he demonstrates a funny walk. Rob was going to have to live with this situation, and ignore some comments and stares that he would inevitably encounter from here on. After all, with his sometimes-uncontrollable sense of humour, he could well have been on the other side regarding this matter. If anything, I believe that Rob's sense of humour heightened after his injury, and that is why I shall be including some specific stories to demonstrate this in chapter five. I'm certain they will make you smile.

4

Going forward

The early part of 1991 was very difficult for Rob. He was coming to terms with his disability, and working extremely hard, to achieve the best possible, physical capabilities, given the nature of his problems. Mornings were particularly bad, when his body was stiff from spasticity, and the first thing he did, was an exercise routine to free up his ankles, and back muscles. I had made him a wobble board that he would stand on, to rock from side to side. Rob had described how he had used a wobble board at the Rehab Unit in Sheffield, to improve his walking. I found some spare timber in the garage, and between us, we came up with a design similar to what Rob had described. This proved very successful in freeing off numerous sets of muscles, thus preparing him for the day ahead. The Rehab Unit had explained to Rob, that the purpose of a wobble board was to reflect the process of walking, and its primary function, was to train his back muscles to relax on one side, whilst tense on the other. It was also beneficial in stopping him throwing his legs out to the side, and snapping his knees back, when he walked. The chief cause of this was that following his injury, his backside was too far back, when he walked, and the wobble board helped by bringing it back into a more normal position.

Rob decided that he wished to pay something back to the head injury unit at the Royal Hallamshire Hospital, and after making some enquiries, it was decided that the best way to do this was to organise a raffle, under the control of a registered charity. We made some enquiries, and set up the charity. I became chairman of the fund, with our next-door neighbour, kindly agreeing to be an appointed trustee. We thought the easiest way to raise some cash, was to organise a one off raffle, and aim to sell a designated number of tickets.

The charity was named 'Bob Pownall's support for 'Neuorcare,' and it was registered with Bassetlaw District Council, under section five of the Lotteries and Amusements Act 1976. Registration number 439. For anyone unfamiliar with this fundraising activity, and seeking to do something similar, it is quite easy to arrange, you simply contact your local district council and they will provide you with the necessary forms that have to be completed. You establish the charity for a limited validity period only, allowing you sufficient time to sell all the tickets, and then you are required to provide the council with an audited set of accounts.

We invited family and friends to donate prizes, and then we had 1,000 x 50 pence tickets printed. Most pleasingly, they were all sold in no time at all, and it was great to see Rob back on the head injury ward, this time presenting a Neurocare cheque in the sum of £500. There was a welcoming party to meet Rob, including a senior nursing sister, plus a number of nurses who had been so professional and supportive during Rob's stay at the Royal Hallamshire Hospital. Neurocare is a fantastic charity, providing all manner of specialised equipment for head injury units. £500 doesn't sound a lot in today's money, but I suppose twenty years ago, it was something Rob should have been very proud of. The draw for the raffle prizes was held on Saturday 30th March 1991, at the offices of the Worksop Trader.

Rob's ongoing problems were many-fold, but obtaining comfortable and functional shoes, was something that he had to pay particular attention to. They had to have cushion soles to counter the over sensitivity of his feet, and they needed to be replaced regularly, as the front of the soles would wear out very quickly, due to his feet sloping downwards. From hereon, Rob would have to be extremely careful not to trip over, due to the contact angle of his shoes, with the ground. This problem was obviously exacerbated whenever he was walking on an uneven surface, or the ground was slippery.

He continued to eat large amounts of food which his body still required as part of the overall recuperating, and healing process. This in itself brought another problem, as he began gaining excessive body weight. He continued to work hard each day, conducting regular exercises, all aimed at improving his physical fitness, and increasing his mobility.

Rob's eyesight suffered as a result of his injury, leaving him with double vision. Fortunately his optician was able to rectify this, and yet another problem had been overcome.

One of Rob's main objectives was to return to driving, but that seemed a long way off, and it was even doubtful whether he would ever drive again. His shiny new Ford Escort car was tucked away in next door's garage, but it remained an incentive for him to continue working hard, for better things to come.

Like the majority of young people, Rob had taken out finance to purchase his new car, and being a responsible individual, he had obtained insurance protection, so that in the event of him being unable to work, and not meet the monthly repayments, the insurance would cover his commitments. The insurance protection was for a maximum period of twelve months, should he become unable to work as a result of redundancy, sickness, or an accident. The policy schedule did clearly state that the insurer would not pay out if the driver of the vehicle had been partaking in the use of alcohol or drugs. That was understandable, and perfectly reasonable, if the claim was against an accident whilst Rob had been driving his car. In Rob's case, the accident occurred, whilst he was socialising with his friends, and had nothing to do with the car, whatsoever.

We made a claim in the belief that the insurer would meet the terms of the insurance contract, without any quibble. Rob and I were very annoyed, when the insurance company refused to pay out, because he had been drinking alcohol prior to the accident. I remember mentioning this situation to the senior consultant looking after Rob at the Royal Hallamshire Hospital, and he said "Tell them from me that he could have suffered the same injury, had he have been drinking lemonade."

I challenged the insurance company, and felt very aggrieved as it was putting the family under additional strain, and I guess Rob was not back to full strength at fighting his own battles. I studied the schedule of the policy, and decided to challenge the insurer through the small claims court. This followed months of wrangling, and whilst Rob was still meeting the payments, we felt he was being cheated out of the protection insurance, which was rightfully his. The summons was issued and a few days later, I received a telephone call from a firm of solicitors, who advised me that they were acting on behalf of the insurance company. A lady asked if I would grant them another ten days, during which they could further investigate the case. I hesitated for a moment, and then I said, "What give you another ten days to find more reasons why Rob should not receive what he was entitled to?" At that, she closed the conversation, and then within the hour, she telephoned me again to say that a cheque would be in the post for the full amount of the arrears.

You have to stand up for your rights in these matters, and not allow big institutions to walk all over you. I had a clear conscience about this matter as Rob, having had a drink of beer prior to his accident, had no bearing upon his insurance claim. This has not been my only experience of insurance companies doing their very best to avoid meeting a claim. I know of people who admit to making false/fraudulent claims, which have been honoured in full. If you are completely honest, sometimes you lose out. This may seem unfair, but honesty is always the best policy, and you have to accept that insurance companies are always aware of potential fraudsters, and that's why they appear to resist paying out without a fight. You have to take on the challenge and be prepared to use whatever legal resources are available.

Rob felt he needed to make a decision over his car, and as sad as it was at the time, he decided that it should go. It was uncertain whether he would get his licence back, and at what stage he would be able to return to his work. I can clearly recall the day when the guy came to collect the car from next door's garage. Although Rob showed no emotion whatsoever, when he stood at our front window, and watched it go up the road. Pat and I were choked, and amazed at Rob's self control, in what was such a sad situation.

On one of Rob's regular visits to see Mr Dias, the surgeon who had operated on him, Rob was asked what he thought about coming off the medication, prescribed to prevent him having epileptic seizures, following his major head surgery. Mr Dias explained that it would be Rob's decision, and he had two choices. He could either remain on these drugs for the rest of his life, or alternatively, he could be slowly weaned off them, and should he have an epileptic seizure, then he would have to return to the drugs indefinitely. Rob was asked to go away and think about it, however Mr Dias did say that should Rob decide to come off the drugs, and he didn't suffer any problems with a seizure, his quality of life would be considerably enhanced. He said it was all down to the Almighty, and if he decided Rob should have a seizure, then it would happen. On the other hand, he might decide that Rob would be seizure free, and it would be all down to him. I remember thinking that was an unusual thing for a doctor to say to his patient, but I wasn't critical, after all, how could anyone criticise a surgeon who had saved your son's life.

Mr Dias then asked Rob about smoking and drinking, and when Rob admitted that he was partaking in both, Mr Dias said, "Robert you must not smoke or drink. With your condition, drinking two pints of beer will have the same effects on you as if your father had drunk five pints." Rob responded by saying, "If I can't smoke and I can't drink, you are not leaving a lot of opportunities for my pleasure, and enjoyment," to which Mr Dias just gave a big smile.

When we had spoken to Rob's GP about Rob going overseas on holiday, he had suggested that it would not be wise for him to travel in an aircraft, due to fluctuations in air pressure, within the confines of the passenger cabin. As we were finishing our consultation with Mr Dias, I expressed my disappointment that on doctor's orders, Rob should avoid travelling in an aeroplane. Mr Dias responded by saying, "I don't agree with what his doctor advised, and I would suggest that it would be perfectly all right for Rob to fly, as long as you don't allow him to pilot the plane!" I asked about Rob's anti-convulsive drugs, and how we would go on entering a different time zone. He suggested that I make up a chart, and gradually alter the intervals between his medications, until he was used to the regional time changes. We went away, and Rob decided to think about his medication for a while, and in the meantime, Pat and I suggested that it might be a good idea for the three of us to take a holiday in Florida, where the warm sunshine would be good for Rob's ongoing recovery.

We booked three tickets to Orlando, and upon our return, Rob would make a decision, whether to come off the anti convulsive medication. Another problem for Rob was difficulty in passing water in public places, and although he would be private within the aircraft toilet, he felt he still might have some problems. We had discussed this with Mr Dias, and he said it would take time, but this phenomenon should go away in due course. He made the obvious suggestion that Rob should go without liquids prior to the flight.

Our flight to Orlando included a scheduled refuelling stop at Bangor Main. We boarded the aircraft at Manchester, and shortly after take off, they began serving breakfast. I then detected some concerned expressions on the faces of the cabin attendants, and then I saw one of them reach for a large white box with a green cross on it. There then followed an announcement from the flight deck asking if there was a doctor on board. They abandoned serving breakfast, and I could see that there was every likelihood that we should be turning round, and heading back to Manchester. There was another announcement from the flight deck, this time asking whether there was anyone on board, who had received any kind of medical training. There was no favourable response to this request, so the captain then informed us that there was a very sick person on board, and he had no alternative but to land at the most convenient airport. He explained that the aircraft was far too heavy to land, and he would have to jettison 30 tons of aviation fuel, before it would be safe to touch down. He informed us how this would happen, and as you would expect, there is a set procedure for the potentially dangerous dumping, of such a large amount of highly flammable, aviation fuel. You can imagine what would likely happen if they were to just let it go. I can see the possibility of a skipper on the bridge of his ship, smoking his pipe, when it started to rain high-octane fuel.

Our captain described how the plane would have to descend below the cloud layer, and then circle an area of the Irish Sea, ensuring that there were no shipping or small boats in the area, before discharging the fuel. The whole process took quite some time, and from where we were sitting, we could see the fuel cascading out of a dump valve, at the rear of the aircraft. Having jettisoned the excess fuel, we were informed that we were going to land at Shannon in the Republic of Ireland, rather than return to Manchester. Apparently, an elderly gentleman had been taken ill soon after take off, and with no medically trained persons onboard the aircraft, the captain had no alternative, but to make an emergency landing.

On the tarmac at Shannon, we had to remain on the aircraft for what seemed an awful long time. We were informed that there was a great deal of paperwork to be completed, and we all had to remain seated, with our seat belts unfastened, whilst the aircraft was being re-fuelled. When eventually, we were clear to go, the estimated flight time from Shannon to Bangor Main, was longer than it had been originally from Manchester to Bangor Main.

Rob was already looking rather tired, and we were concerned about how he would now stand up to the long journey ahead. He kept his intake of liquid to a minimum, and we implemented the re-scheduling of his medication. We continued adjusting the times when he took the tablets, and apart from extreme tiredness, Rob seemed to be handling things very well. Before we finally landed in Orlando, the captain gave the latest news about the sick gentleman that we had dropped off in Shannon. He said the man had received surgery for appendicitis, and he was now recovering nicely in hospital. I still can't get my head round how someone could be taken so ill within a few minutes after take off. Something like a heart attack may be, but appendicitis is something else, and I guess the man had probably been in trouble, before boarding the plane at Manchester.

We eventually landed in Orlando, and we were all very relieved when we arrived at our hotel. We stayed at the Lake Buena Vista resort for our first week, and St Petersburg on the west coast, for the second week. St Petersburg was an ideal location, where our hotel was in close proximity to the famous St Petersburg beach. Rob and I spent a lot of time in the lovely warm sea, and the exercise from swimming, was excellent therapy for Rob's mobility problems. It was our first holiday following Rob's injury and we all returned the better for it.

Before Rob's accident, he was a good golfer with loads of natural ability. He had a nice set of clubs, and golf was one of his favourite pastimes. Now that he was slowly getting around on his feet, he began wondering if golf might still be a possibility. Obviously, he would never be able to walk the length of a full golf course, but if he could still hit a reasonable ball, and manage around the greens, a golf cart could be used to transport him around. We decided to visit nearby Kilton golf course, just to see how he could swing a club. Rob set up a ball, and with one of his woods, he took a full swing. Unfortunately, he missed the ball, spun round on his feet, and fell to the ground. I took one look at him and I said "Rob I think your golfing days are over." He saw the funny side, and together, we had a jolly good laugh. I know it was only one ball, but comparing him then, to how he could play before his injury, my advice was to give it up, and focus on something else more suited to his changed circumstances. I personally don't subscribe to those people who attempt to climb Everest in a wheel chair, or go to the South Pole on crutches. Whilst I do admire their courage, and determination, I believe that there are many other pursuits to be undertaken, that are less stressful, and well within their restricted physical capabilities.

It was now approaching the first anniversary of Rob's accident, and whilst he was still struggling with his walking, he was thinking about returning to work. His employer Great Mills (DIY) had been very supportive, and whilst he was only paid for a few months of his absence from work, they had very kindly kept his position open, should he eventually wish to return to their employment. Rob had a meeting with his old boss, and it was agreed that he should return to his previous job, initially on a part-time basis. He started back just before the Christmas holidays, and Pat and I were very concerned, as we knew it would be really tough for him, and now more than twelve months since his injury, we wondered how much further progress, could realistically be achieved.

In the summer of 1992, the three of us took another holiday, this time to the Greek Island of Rhodes. Our next-door neighbour Jack Stewart had recommended the resort of Falaraki, having passed through the place during a recent holiday in Rhodes Town. It was a last minute affair, and I didn't bother doing any research. We found a small family run apartment and thought it would be fine. We were a long way back from the centre of Falaraki, and Rob had great difficulty getting about, particularly in the evenings, when we had to go into town for the restaurants. We used taxis wherever we could, but still Rob was struggling to walk, just short distances.

The US navy was in town, coming ashore from the aircraft carrier USS George Washington. The sailors were crazy guys, and their behaviour in the streets of Falaraki was unbelievable. Having served in the Merchant Navy as an engineering officer, I couldn't get over how their military police should allow them to use such bad language in a public place. If we had been found behaving as badly as that, we would have been locked up, with the keys thrown away. Clearly, Rob was on holiday with his parents under considerable sufferance, but his opportunities to get away by alternative means were very limited. We all tried to make the best of the situation, and at least it took Rob away from his working environment for a short time, thereby giving his body a well- earned period of rest.

As far as Rob was concerned, he was determined to make a full and complete recovery, but as his parents, Pat and I were somewhat sceptical. We both believed that although his achievements since the injury had been a blessing and incredible, we thought any further improvements, were unlikely to happen.

Back at work, Rob was struggling; he would come home exhausted and looked physically drained, with severe spasticity showing in his face. He would tell us that after only one hour at work, he felt drained of energy, and it was a struggle to make his legs go. I remember one day when Pat and I visited the store, we observed Rob obviously struggling to walk about, and it caused us considerable concern. Whilst I admired his determination to get back to physical work, I could see that it was causing him severe discomfort, and strain. Pat and I worried continuously about the situation, but no matter what we said to Rob, he was adamant that he would continue with his work. Slowly we could see the strength draining from him, and we were very concerned that he might become ill, or suffer another accident, as life at work was becoming more challenging.

Another year passed by, and Pat and I decided that we needed to get Rob away for a good rest, and take another holiday. For some reason, Rob had decided to have what I considered to be a silly hair cut. To me it looked as if he had received a short back and sides, whilst having a basin on his head. I thought he looked ridiculous, and with his awkward walking, I thought he was attracting unnecessary attention to himself. At the airport, I could see people looking at Rob, as I guess they were wondering what was causing him to walk in such a strange manner.

We were pleased with our apartment, but the topography of the surrounding area was rather hilly, and Rob had considerable difficulty walking around, still unable to walk comfortably in trainers, or light shoes. Stress levels were high on that holiday, as I was not pleased about Rob's appearance, and I didn't think he was presenting himself to the world, as he should. He had put on some weight, and his choice of cloths did not make him look as smart, as I thought he could be. It all culminated in one of those enormous rows that every family experience from time to time. We had been to a bar for a lunchtime drink, and after two pints of Guinness, strong stuff, I must admit, Rob's walking was dreadful. When we arrived back at our apartment, things blew up and I guess we all said things we shouldn't. When it was all over, Rob agreed to let me cut his hair, and whilst he sat in a chair on the balcony, I gave him a smart trim, using Pat's nail scissors. I was very relieved about this, and in my eyes as well as Pat's, he looked more like the Rob we knew before his accident.

Following our argument, I suggested to Rob that in my opinion it was time that he faced up to the reality of his disability, otherwise life would prove impossible, and he would be very miserable. I applauded his determination to get back to full strength, but it was obvious prior to this holiday, that work was becoming almost impossible to keep up with. I suggested that when we return from this holiday, we would seek some advice and find out what options would be available, by way of financial support, and benefits. We contacted the local authorities, and we had a meeting with a guy in Worksop, who suggested that Rob should become registered as being disabled. I think this was a bitter pill for Rob to swallow, but it's no use making yourself very unhappy by attempting to achieve the impossible. Rob was advised to apply for the mobility element of the disability living allowance, and also to apply to Remploy regarding the status of his employment. Remploy interviewed Rob, and decided to take him on their books. He would still work for Great Mills, but Remploy would pay his wages, thus taking some pressure off Rob's levels of performance.

Life was not getting any easier for Rob, and the pressures were showing. I thought he should consider a new job, which was less demanding physically, and one that would make better use of his considerable intelligence. After all, we had always known that Rob had a high intelligent quotient, which was discovered at an early age. He was attending primary school at the time when we were living in Leicester, and one day Pat and I were invited to a meeting with Rob's teacher. We were informed that they were not happy about his progress at school, and asked our permission to conduct some intelligence tests. Naturally, as parents, we were somewhat concerned, and disappointed about this, but decided that it was in Rob's best interest to get to the route of these apparent problems. We returned to school, where the teacher explained that the results had shown Rob to have an IQ well above average, and they wished to repeat the tests to make sure they had got it right. The tests were repeated, and the original result was confirmed. They then decided that Rob was bored in class, and needed some additional challenges, in order to maintain his interest. This happened, and much later on in his education he went on to achieve very good 'O' & 'A' level results in his GSE examinations. Knowing all this, Pat and I thought Rob should be in a job that would task his brain, rather than his body.

By now, what Rob really needed, was to get his driving licence reinstated, and to this end, he contacted his GP, who gave the go ahead for Rob to re-apply for his licence. Rob described how the doctor held a rule between Rob's separated fore finger and thumb, and then released the rule, which Rob should attempt to grasp between his finger and thumb. He passed this test with flying colours, and according to the doctor, Rob's reactions were above average, for this kind of test. It was now 12 months since Rob came off the anti-convulsive drugs, and thankfully he had not had a problem. He was now able to re-apply for the reinstating of his driving licence, and thankfully his application was successful.

Rob was never one to mess around, and one evening when we returned home from work, there was a strange car parked on the drive. Rob had been out during the day, and purchased a second hand Austin Maestro, that turned out to be a liability. It was in poor condition, and became a drain on his limited resources. Pat and I were very unhappy about this situation, and suggested to Rob that he should consider getting a much better car. He agreed to let us look around, to see what offers might be available on new vehicles. We found a very good deal on a new Fiat Uno, and once again, Rob had got a car that he could be proud of.

Having been advised by a representative of the local authority to apply for the mobility element of the 'Disability Living Allowance', Rob proceeded with the application. It wasn't necessarily for then, but for the years to come. I remember when he was still a patient in Lodge Moor Hospital; a senior nurse told me that Rob would have problems later on, with his back and knees, basically, from wear and tear, due to the enormous effort he would have to put in, to simply walk around. He completed the comprehensive application forms, and they were sent off for consideration. In my heart of hearts, I never doubted that his application would be anything other than successful. Having carefully studied the forms, I couldn't see how he could not meet the strict criteria for a successful claim.

Several weeks later, Rob received a letter from the DSS (Department of Social Security) to inform him that his application had been rejected, on the grounds that his disabilities were not severe enough for him to be awarded the mobility allowance. We were very disappointed with this decision, but we had the right to an appeal. I decided that I would assume responsibility to represent and support Rob, through the appeal process. Once again, there were pages of forms to be completed, plus a detailed submission on my part, as to why I believed he should be awarded this important allowance. It was not just Rob's walking that was proving very difficult, he was always in danger of tripping, which was evident from the way he was wearing his shoes out, due to excessive wear to the front of the soles. The spasticity in Rob's face was an ongoing problem. It manifested itself more so whenever the weather was cold, or if he became stressed.

We were given a date for the appeal, and we had to attend a tribunal in Mansfield. As we sat in the waiting room, it was evident that the majority of appeal claimants were elderly and most seemed to be in very poor health. I sat there thinking that compared with some of these poorly folk, Rob didn't seem to have much of a chance. Most of the other individuals appealing over a claim rejection were either represented by a health care representative, or a social worker.

We had to wait a long time, but eventually it was our turn, and we were called into a room, where the hearing would take place. There were three men sat behind a bench, plus a lady representative from the DSS (Department of Social Security), who sat along side us, and it was her role to defend the decision that Rob's claim should not be granted. Regarding the three men who would rule on our appeal, the one sat in the middle was a barrister, the one on his left was a doctor, and the one on his right, was a union representative, viewing the case from a disability perspective. The DSS lady was initially asked to justify why

Rob's claim had been rejected, and then the questioning from the bench was directed at us. Following a few questions to Rob, the doctor began asking me to elaborate on Rob's disability, and how it was affecting his daily life. He asked about his mother's role in all this, which I suggested, was considerable. He accepted this, and commented about the amount of spasticity showing in Rob's face.

Prior to the tribunal, Rob and I agreed that we should not exaggerate anything and Rob refused to use a walking stick, as he had entered the room. As things progressed, I began having doubts about our chances of success, as the DSS representative seemed to me to be winning the argument. Following questions from each member of the appeal panel, the barrister said he was going to adjourn, whilst they discussed Rob's case in private. Together with the DSS representative, we were asked to return to the waiting room, until called again. Several minutes later, we were summoned back into the appeal room, and once again, invited to take a seat. The barrister addressed Rob, and said they had a problem. They had considered the case very carefully, and wished to reverse the DSS decision of rejection. However, he said, there are two levels of benefit, and due to some of the wording recorded on the appeal claim form, they would not be able to grant him, the maximum benefit.

The barrister asked Rob to look through the window, and view a supermarket on the other side of the road. He said to Rob "How would you feel if you walked from here to the supermarket unaided." Rob replied, that his legs would be tired, which I knew to be the case. Rob was then informed that he had been granted the full benefit, which came as a great relief. The barrister and the doctor, then stood up to shake our hands, and to our surprise, the union representative pushed back a wheel chair and gave us a rye smile. We would never have guessed that he was disabled.

Rob struggled on to keep his fulltime job working for Great Mills until 1996. Looking back, Rob describes these years as the period, where most things including work, were in a state of limbo.

Pat and I needed a holiday, just the two of us to get away and relax. We booked up and off we went, once again to Tenerife. It gave us much opportunity to discuss Rob and his future, and we spent at lot of time thinking about what he might do to earn a decent living, in a job that would be better suited to his physical disabilities.

We telephoned Rob, and I suggested that a sales job in financial services might be an idea, at least something for him to think about. Accessing certain properties with steps and stairs might be a problem, but I considered he might get more job satisfaction from that kind of career, rather than a full time desk job. Working in a DIY store was too physically demanding, and if something different didn't come along very soon, we were fearful that Rob might crack up. Many a person would have settled for state benefits, rather than struggle to work as Rob was doing. His determination and courage were to be admired, but we could detect signs that Rob was running out of steam. Typical of Rob, not being one to waste time, as soon as we arrived home from our holiday he announced that he had secured an interview with the Prudential Insurance Company, for a position in sales. His application was successful, and he was soon turning out in a smart blue suit and carrying his new brief case.

We converted our fourth bedroom into an office from where he completed his paperwork, and made his customer appointments. It made me smile, because rather than sit in his home office in his casual cloths, he would be dressed as if he was going to visit a customer. There was a lot of study involved in this new role, and Rob had to pass his financial planning examinations, to keep his job, and comply with the regulations of the industry.

Those exams were very tough, and I'm sure Rob will agree that his mother played a major roll in supporting him through endless hours of revision. She often used to say that she was now capable of passing those examinations herself. There were endless amounts of things to remember, and they spent many hours together, going through mock exam papers, until he reached the necessary pass levels. We were very proud that Rob successfully passed his financial planning examinations, FP1, FP2 & FP3.

Rob enjoyed the job, and proved to be successful with his level of sales. He worked with a great bunch of guys, and he was going from strength to strength. Unfortunately the Prudential were going through some restructuring, and Rob and all his colleagues were made redundant. He managed to find similar employment and went on to study for other qualifications including, CF2, CF7, CF9 & C Map. He also passed Securities Level Two, which qualified him to deal in stocks and shares. Rob worked for a number of insurance companies, and turned in very successful sales. However, it was always a great strain on him physically, particularly during the wintertime, when both his legs and back were tight, and awkward to move.

In 1998, Rob made a decision to move from our family home and he purchased a small house in his hometown of Worksop. This gave him far more independence, which was obviously what he required. He was now in a good job, buying his own property, and things were looking up. Having said this, he still had to work at maintaining his physical fitness, and walking was not getting any easier. He had many types of exercising apparatus, including a treadmill, rowing machine, weights, and an exercise bench.

Rob always had a passion for motorcycles, for which I probably have to take full responsibility. It all started when we were collecting our pet dog Flossy from a nearby kennels, and as we were waiting for her I noticed there was an old Moped lying on the ground. Rob would have been about 12 years of age at the time, and when the lady came to us with Flossy I asked her about the Moped, and she said we were welcome to take it away. We bundled it into the car, and took it home, where upon, I suggested to Rob that we strip it down to the very last nut and bolt, and then restore it. Over the following months it proved an interesting exercise, and when we finally got it back together again, it provided great pleasure when we started the engine. We had that Moped for years, and very often, Rob would ask me to take it to a nearby private lane, where he would ride it up and down. It kept him amused, but Pat was not happy about this, and she said I was encouraging him to ride motorbikes. Sure enough, as soon as he became sixteen years old, he bought himself a motorbike. A small one to begin with, and progressively he exchanged them for more powerful models. We had a terrible scare one evening prior to Rob's head injury, when he was knocked off his motorcycle by a speeding police car. We were sat at home waiting for Rob to return from night school, and with the television turned down low, we could usually hear the purring of his 50cc motorcycle, as it approached along our cul-de-sac. This particular evening, it was past the time when he was expected home, and we were becoming rather anxious. The telephone rang, and it was someone informing us that Rob had been involved in an accident. It had happened only a few hundred yards from home, so we ran to where we could see blue flashing lights, and wondered what we were going to find.

There were several police cars at the scene, and just as we approached, they were closing the doors of an ambulance. A policeman said to Pat, "If you are the mother, you can travel with him in the ambulance, if you wish". She leapt into the back of the vehicle, and it sped off towards Bassetlaw District Hospital. I won't go through all the details of what transpired, because it left a nasty taste in my mouth, as to how it was handled both by the CPS (Crown

Prosecution Service), and the Nottinghamshire Constabulary.

The accident occurred at a junction, where Rob had signalled to make a right hand turn. As he approached the centre of the road, and about to make the turn, a police car travelling at high speed struck him. Apparently it had been giving chase to a stolen motorcycle, and was not displaying any lights whatsoever, not even sidelights, never mind flashing warning lights, despite it being within the hours of darkness. The highly powered police patrol car, had been speeding in a 30 mph area, and without showing any lights, it was a miracle that Rob had not been killed. Clearly to me the police officer driving the car was breaking the law, and should have been called to account. The offence was investigated, and I was informed three months later that the CPS had decided not to bring a case against the officer driving the police car, and that the Nottinghamshire Constabulary, had decided not to invoke their disciplinary procedures. I was not impressed with those decisions, but having taken legal advice, I was persuaded to put the matter to the back of my mind. My solicitor said I should need a great deal of money, and in his opinion, I would be fighting an impossible case. It seems that the police can be above the law in this type of situation. Fortunately, Rob was not seriously injured, just bruising to his body, and I guess, his pride.

He lost the no claims bonus on his insurance, although he was the innocent party, and he had to replace his new leather jacket, that was torn in the accident. Overall it cost him a lot of money, as well as some considerable pain, and whilst he was in hospital and then recovering at home, he didn't receive one single call from the police, to enquire about his state of health. I was not impressed.

Now ten years on from Rob's head injury, Rob decided to have another motorbike, despite Pat and I doing our best to persuade him otherwise. I used to worry about him out on the road with a motorcycle, before his head injury, but now with spasticity in his legs, I wondered how he would control the thing. Remarkably, he managed extremely well, and despite the worry, I was very impressed when I saw him shoot off up the road on a very sporty looking machine. He had several bikes; all sports models, capable of very high speed. On one occasion as I arrived home from an overseas business trip, I was asked to look inside the garage. To my surprise, there was a BMW 100RS motorbike that Rob had bought for me. It was a very kind gesture, but I soon realised that I was not going to be a really confident, born again motorcyclist. It was too heavy for me, so not to be beaten, he then bought me a 900cc GPZ, which was a beast of a machine, but a great deal lighter than the BMW. I used to ride both machines, but never felt particularly relaxed or confident. One Sunday morning, I nearly fell off the GPZ, and that was the end of my motorcycling.

The years passed by, and Rob's career in the financial services sector continued despite a number of set backs due to restructuring within the industry. Many of the large insurance companies were having redundancies within their field sales teams, and Rob was unfortunately affected by this strategy. Following several redundancies, he had to find alternative employment, but it was becoming increasingly difficult, with the physical effects of walking being more apparent, and jobs in the market place, in steep decline.

In 2010 Rob was married to Ann, whose first husband had died under tragic circumstances. They have two children from Ann's previous marriage, Lewis and Lauren, and the family reside in Ann's hometown of Leigh in Lancashire, together with their two dogs, Beau and Tink, plus three cats, Milo, Shadow and Oscar.

Rob's wedding was a wonderful occasion, and Lewis made a very moving speech, that we shall always remember.

Rob waited a long time to find the right partner, but thankfully it was well worth it. He is now very settled and Pat and I are so pleased that he has the family life that he greatly deserves. We trust they will have a long and happy life together.

5

Rob's Humour

Rob's profile

I have not found it easy writing about Rob's unfortunate head injury, and the long journey back, after his life saving surgery. I find it much easier writing about things pleasant and amusing. However, I am pleased that I finally got round to finishing something that I have been contemplating, for a long time. Now that the worst has already been told, I wanted to include a very different chapter that illustrates Rob's true nature, and in particular, his great sense of humour. He has a way with him that involves things sometimes going a little awry, or perhaps, not quite the way he'd planned. He's very capable of sticking up for his rights, and does not suffer fools gladly. Poor levels of service and discourtesy are amongst his 'pet hates.'

Rob is very interested in cooking, and has the required culinary skills to prepare some excellent food. He and I have shared many great experiences together, some of which are detailed in my other books 'Funny How Things Work Out' and 'Onwards and Upwards'. We have a very good father/son relationship, and I consider us to be great mates. He has excellent IT skills, and whenever I get into difficulty with my computer, he is my first point of contact.

I trust that some of the following stories will portray Rob's true character, and at the same time, engender the occasional smile.

Watch where you're going with that bike

I recall one Sunday afternoon, when Rob was in his early teens. He had been out on his new drop handle bar sports bicycle, and was returning home to Hemmingfield Rise. I spotted him pushing his bike up the road, and wondered why he was not riding it. He came into the house in a bit of a fluster, and then cracked up in hysterical laughter. "What's happened?" I said. He regained some self-control, and then explained how he had been riding his bicycle along Hemmingfield Rise when for some reason; he was looking down at the Derailleur gear mechanism instead of paying attention to what was ahead of him. He steered the bike into the front of a neighbour's parked car, and found himself sprawled across the bonnet of a nice new Ford Focus. He jumped off the car bonnet, and grabbed his bike from the road, then hurried round the corner to return home as quickly as possible. We did go and check that he had not caused any damage to the neighbour's car and fortunately it was only Rob's pride that had taken a dent.

New Year's Eve party

Rob had been invited to attend a New Years Eve party by one of his mates, and after a couple of drinks too many, Rob thought he should say a few words, following the chimes of midnight, from Big Ben. In Rob's words, "Not the best thing he's ever done." Rob was handed his coat by his mate's father, who then, politely asked Rob to leave. Without going into too much detail, Rob had expressed some strong desires towards his mate's sister, and was promptly given his marching orders. The following day Rob thought it appropriate that he should visit the house again, to deliver a formal apology to his mate's parents. His mate's mother said "Not to worry Rob, as another guest had stayed the night, and he had been shouting and banging on the bedroom wall. "If this wasn't bad enough," she said, "He had wet the bed and ruined the mattress."

Rob reckons the morale to this story is - It's all right making a fool of yourself, provided someone does something much worse!

Purchasing a CD

For some reason, Rob was not in a particularly good mood as he visited the local supermarket to purchase a CD. The CD was entitled 'Best of the 1980s and when he returned to his car, he thought he would make sure that it worked ok. CDs one and two played fine, but he was not a happy bunny, when he discovered that the third one wouldn't play. He went back into the store, and complained at the customer services desk, in a rather abrupt manner. When he arrived home he tried the replacement CDs in his music system, and he was not best pleased, when he found that CDs one and two were fine, but again, the third one, would not work. He was now in a really bad mood, and returning to the store once again, he asked to see the manager. When the manager arrived, Rob said, "What kind of rubbish are you selling here?" The manager looked very carefully at the CD set, and said, "No wonder CD three won't play, it's a karaoke DVD."

Whoops Rob, you made a right boo boo there!

Christmas dinner

Although Rob has become an excellent cook, it was not always the case.

Following his injury, and when he had re-located to his own property, he decided to abandon the traditional Christmas dinner at our family home, and invite a few guests to his place. He went to a great deal of effort to prepare what he hoped would be an excellent meal. All was going well, until it came to preparing the stuffing. He emptied the contents from a Paxo bag into a dish, and put it in the microwave oven. Had he read the instructions properly; he would have seen that you have to add water!!

The consequences of micro waving dry stuffing mix were lots of sparks, followed by a rich blue flame. He opened the microwave oven door, grabbed the plate, and threw it out of the kitchen window, into the garden.

From the lounge he heard a voice say "Dinner's going well then?" to which Rob curtly replied "Cook your own f****** dinner then."

Rob's flying skills

I originally recorded this story in my memoirs entitled 'Funny How Things Work Out', but thought it was worthy of being included in this chapter as in my opinion it indicates the type of guy Rob is. He has a distinctive character that developed at an early age.

When Rob was about ten years of age, he asked if he could have a model aircraft for Christmas, one that you build from a kit, and it must have radio controls.

We visited a model shop in Doncaster, made a purchase, and the man in the shop said "Don't try to fly this plane until you have had some lessons." He gave me a telephone number, and asked me to give him a call, when we were ready to fly.

I have always taken the bull by the horns, and instead of reading about the techniques of flying model aircraft, and how the radio controls are operated, I went full speed ahead and believed we knew sufficient to get us started. Having finished the building process, we were now in possession of a splendid looking model aeroplane. I telephoned the man at the shop, and he invited us to join him at a field near to Doncaster, where he was a member of a model-flying club. He asked us to meet him at a certain time, and he would then give us some flying instruction.

Whilst I had been building the plane, I had noticed a small rectangular shaped orange flag attached to the radio antenna. There was a number 32 on the flag, and I didn't know what this meant, nor did I see any reason to find out.

On the day of the flying lesson, Rob and I loaded the plane in the back of our estate car, and we made our way to Doncaster. Arriving at the field, there was an aerobatic model in German wartime livery, looping the loop, and completing many impressive manoeuvres. We got out of the car, and I opened the tailgate to access the plane. The radio controls were laid by the side of the plane, and Rob being Rob, flicked the activating switch to the on position. All of a sudden, this splendid model aeroplane, performing miraculous barrel rolls etc, fell from the sky and smashed into the ground. It was totally wrecked, and the pilot shouted "No one is on 32"and then it registered with me, what the number 32 signified. There in front of us, was a post with a large board attached, and written in chalk on this board, was the number 32. It obviously showed the frequency on which the plane in the air was operating on, thereby warning all others using the same frequency, to keep their controls switched off.

In a state of shock and panic, I put our plane back into the car, and said "Rob get into the car quick." "Why dad?" he asked, "We've only just arrived." "Get in the car now," I said, "I'll explain to you later what this is all about." Rob looked very bemused, but I guess my facial expression indicated that all was not well, and once inside the car, we drove away at high speed. Whether they realised it was us that caused the crash, I shall never know, but for sure, I didn't contact that shop owner, ever again.

Not sure what to do next, I decided to get a book on the principles of flight, applicable to flying model aircraft. I thought that if I could understand the basics, we could start off on our own, and get better with experience.

It is very difficult to fly model aircraft, particularly the one like ours, which was a high performance, fast moving plane. It's easy enough taking off, but then you have to start a turn, before it gets out of range from the radio signals. As you turn and when the plane is coming back towards you, the hand controls are reversed, and if you are not careful, you can easily lose control. You've guessed it, that's exactly what happened on our maiden flight. I was at the controls, and things went belly up, with the plane crashing into a nearby field of cabbages. We scooped up all the fragmented bits and started a process of rebuilding the damn thing. I crashed it again, and repeated the building process; this time building two sets of wings and fuselages.

For our third attempt at flying, Rob had persuaded me that he should have go. Pat wished to accompany us to a nearby-disused airfield, and all the pre-flight preparations were completed. Rob is left-handed, and he seemed very awkward in his handling of the controls.

We started the engine, and lined the plane up along a nice stretch of concrete runway. I went over the take off procedure again, and again, making it very clear to Rob that once the plane had reached maximum speed, you just pull back very slightly on the elevator, and up she would go.

There was great tension and anticipation as Rob pulled back the throttle, and sure enough, it shot off with great speed. "Pull back on the elevator lever" I said, but nothing happened. "Pull the elevator ," I repeated, but still it was on the ground, and fast approaching one of those wire link sheep fences, which lay straight ahead. I desperately shouted for him to pull on the elevator lever, but it was too late, and the plane shot clean through the fence, smashing it into many pieces. I'm not proud of the fact that I inadvertently, came out with the 'F' word. I could not prevent myself from saying to Rob, "What the f*** were you doing.

Rob was in tears, Pat was appalled at my language in front of our son, and there was all my rebuild work, lying in bits and pieces.

We decided that flying model aircraft was not for us, and I put it all back together with the spare parts, and then sold it for £80. I hope the buyer had better luck than we did!!

Although our model aircraft flying wasn't funny at the time, both Rob and I have had many a good laugh since, and I often picture the scene when we were speeding out of that flying field in Doncaster, having caused such a dreadful disaster. I felt a bit like Mr Bean, only with son!!

Great Mills DIY

During Rob's time at Great Mills DIY in Worksop, both before and following his injury, he often came home with a humorous tale to tell.

They were changing their colour scheme, and as such all fire doors required a repaint. Rob went in one Saturday morning, and was asked to paint the managers office door. Rob carefully removed the door from its hinges, and then carried it into the warehouse, where upon, he leaned it against a wall. As he was walking away to get a paint brush, he heard a dreadful smash, and when he turned round, he was horrified to see that the door had crashed down on the concrete floor, and was now in two pieces.

The self-closing mechanism had hit the floor first, and it had come off, with the top two inches of the door. In a state of shock and embarrassment, Rob took the door outside, and propped it against the wall. He was sweating as he set off to explain to the manager what had happened. He had only walked a few steps, when he heard another loud crack, and to his horror, the wind had blown the door over. Rob walked back, and when he saw the state of the door, he thought 'ohhh heck.' The glass safety panel had collided with a nearby pallet truck, and the glass had shattered into many pieces. The manager's office door was now two inches shorter, with no glass safety panel.

Rob plucked up courage to go and tell the manager what had happened. In Rob's own words he said to the manager "Sir you need to come and look at your door, something has happened." Rob says, "The manager didn't swear, he just looked at me as if to say "Why the f*** did I employ you?"

Practical jokes

There was regular practical joking at the Great Mills store, and one day Rob was asked for the keys to his Mk 2 Ford Escort. They said that a customer had inadvertently locked their car keys into the boot, and it was the same model as Rob's car. Rob thought it was worth a try, and handed over the keys.

That evening as closing time approached, the management informed the staff that there was a new company policy, and they were introducing random security checks on all employees' vehicles. When it came to Rob's turn, he was asked to open his car boot, and to his horror, there was a £200 lawn mower sitting there. Rob had a bit of explaining to do, but it all ended with a good laugh.

Customer enquiries

I shall never forget the day Rob came home from Great Mills, and struggled to stop laughing, to tell me how a guy had asked Rob for some dildo rail!

The paint section

Rob and a colleague were assigned to work on the paint section, which involved clearing all the shelves, and rearranging the racking. The job was about completed, and Rob and his mate were sitting on the floor, admiring their work. Rob's mate said, "One of the racks is slightly out of line," and he promptly stood up, walked to a particular rack, and gave it a kick. Shock of horrors; as the entire racking came crashing down, with paint tins spilling their contents all over the floor. Rob reckons there were over 100 tins of paint destroyed in that incident, and they had to use snow shovels, in the cleaning up operation.

The forklift truck

Rob has two lovely stories about colleagues driving the Great Mills forklift truck.

Rob was asked to work overnight, to accompany the store manager on security duties. When I asked what that was all about, Rob explained that there was a problem with the warehouse shutter door; therefore the building could not be secured properly. The cause of this situation resulted from a fellow worker using the fork lift truck to ease open the roller shutter door, as it was proving difficult to open by hand. He forced the door fully open using the elevated forks of the truck, but unfortunately, he forgot to lower them, before attempting to drive back into the warehouse. The top of the forks hit the opening/closing mechanism, and completely knocked the door off its mounts.

On another occasion, one of Rob's fellow workers had recently passed his driving proficiency test on the forklift truck. He was asked to attend to a delivery lorry, parked in the yard, waiting to be unloaded. He had to lift a pallet from the lorry, and transport it into the warehouse. Unfortunately, as he was manoeuvring the forklift truck in the yard, his safety boot became entangled with a control pedal, and he reversed at great speed crashing backwards through the boundary fence, into the adjacent property. Thankfully, no one was hurt, but you can imagine the laughter that incident created.

Smart arse salesman at Great Mills

Occasionally, they would have guest sales people promoting specific products, and one day, a real spiv arrived to set up a double-glazing promotion, at the entrance to the store. Rob described this guy as a true tosser, wearing light beige trousers, and a bright blue jacket. Rob was working at the customer services desk, when the salesman approached Rob, and asked where the toilets were located. Off went the sales guy to visit the loo, and when he returned a few minutes later, Rob could instantly see that something had changed. As Rob looked closer, he could see that the sales guy had obviously had some water issues, as there was a huge dark patch on the front of his smart beige trousers. Rob couldn't contain himself, and hid behind the customer services desk to have a really good belly laugh.

ATC Worksop

As a young lad, Rob joined the ATC (Royal Air Force - Air Cadets) and regularly came home with some hilarious stories.

He had been on the firing range, receiving instruction on how to safely fire the Lee Enfield .303 rifle. They had been informed, and warned, about the recoil from this powerful weapon, when the trigger was pulled, and to combat this, they had been instructed to pull the butt of the rifle, hard into their shoulder. Rob fired several shots before the instructor ordered him off the range, for shooting with his eyes shut!!

They had been on exercises, and cooking was by means of a portable Esbit stove. Rob had placed the hexane fuel tablets into the stove, but it was quite windy, and he was struggling to get them to ignite. Seeking shelter, he relocated to a nearby structure, under which, he was able to light the cooker. He thought he was doing just fine, until an officer came marching on the scene, and went ballistic. Rob had only lit the stove under a highly flammable fuel store.

Rob's DIY

Rob is the first to admit that he is far better at theory, rather than practical skills.

One Saturday when his mother returned home from work, she shouted to me "What's all this sawdust on the stairs?"

"I don't know," I said, "You had better ask Rob." "Rob," she said, "where has all this saw dust on the staircase come from?" "Haven't got a clue?" He said.

Pat asked Rob what he had been doing, and he explained that he had been fitting a wall bracket in his bedroom, to mount his portable television. When I looked up the staircase, there were several holes where the drill had come straight through the wall. Pat went hairless, and I had to get the ladder from the garage and fill the holes before repairing the decoration.

Soon after Rob's sister Tracey was married, she asked Rob and I if we would assemble a pine kitchen cupboard for her. On the day of this flat pack assembly exercise, Tracey and her husband Ian were out shopping, and Rob and I were left alone to get on with the task.

It was a very nice piece of furniture, and we were progressing really well, when I found some difficulty fitting a wooden dowel peg into a pre-drilled hole. It was very tight, so I asked Rob to pass me the hammer. I tapped it a couple of times to no effect, so I gave it a really good bang. There followed an awful sound of splitting wood, and we were horrified to see that I had split the side of the cabinet.

We both collapsed in laughter and we wondered what we should do. Tracey is very meticulous, and Ian is a quality engineer by profession, so we both knew our repair strategy had to be a good one.

We glued the spit as best we could, but if we looked very carefully, it was there to be seen.

Ian was expected home first so I said to Rob, "When he arrives, what ever you do, don't laugh." You can imagine the tension, Ian arrived, and his first comments were, that he liked the looks of the cabinet. I accidentally caught eye contact with Rob, and he collapsed in laughter. Ian soon twigged that something was wrong, and sure enough, he found where we had attempted to repair the split. We came clean with him, and he was very reasonable about it.

Now the big test was coming as Tracey was expected home any minute. We three agreed that if we were to get away scot-free, we should all have to keep a straight face. In she came, and as soon as she began her critical inspection, Rob cracked up in hysterical laughter.

She spotted the problem, and went ballistic. After some discussion we were let off the hook, because that side of the cabinet was going against a wall, so we survived to tell the tale!

Things aren't much different all those years on. Rob's wife Ann asked him to fit a new door, separating the kitchen from the lounge. The existing one had glass panels, and their two dogs were becoming a regular nuisance.

Whilst confined to the kitchen, they were making noises as they could see the cats in the lounge, through the panels in the glass door.

Rob purchased a solid wooden door, and borrowed all the necessary tools from me, including my recently acquired, electric wood planer. Rob feeling rather professional measured the door against the frame, and began using the electric planer. Ann was complaining, because he was spreading sawdust all around the room. He made three attempts at fitting the door, and then, he had another good burst, with my electric planer. The living room was now looking a bit like a sawdust wonderland.

Rob tried the door once more, and it fitted a treat. Ann who was with Rob in the lounge said, "Its fine, but I can see the kitchen." Rob looked up, and there was a three-inch gap at the top. Ann said "By the way Rob, there's a bag here that you're supposed to attach to the planer, to contain all the sawdust, you silly b***er."

They had to return to the DIY store for another door, which fortunately fitted a treat. So all was well, the second time/door around!

Don't laugh in church

It was the occasion of one of our nephew's wedding, and I had pre-warned Rob that he should behave himself, whilst we were in church for the marriage ceremony. It took place in about 1997 at a church in Staffordshire. My wife Pat, our daughter Tracey, together with her husband Ian and their son Jack, who was about two years old at the time, were also attending this wedding.

Having pre-warned Rob to behave himself in Church, I lectured Ian regarding the same subject, as he too, can be very roughish in this type of situation. I also instructed Rob and Ian to sit apart, so that they wouldn't be able to have eye contact, or whisper to each other.

Arriving at the church, we were ushered to our seats, just a few rows from the front. I purposely sat between Rob and Ian with Tracey and Pat at the other end of the pew, with little Jack sitting between Ian and me.

Little Jack, was finding it difficult to sit still, and began moving along in front of us whilst making the odd comment. For me it was like sitting on a time bomb, because I knew that the slightest innuendo or unusual happening would trigger off Ian and Rob in uncontrollable giggles.

Little Jack came along to my end of the pew, and he passed wind, which was both audible, and detectable by smell.

That was it, and the laughing and embarrassment began. I was sweating, and asked Rob and Ian to be more respectful whilst in church.

We were still sitting down waiting for the service to begin, and I kept digging Rob in his ribs, in an attempt to bring him under control.

I had just settled things down when Jack came along the row again, and said in loud voice "Rob these are my dancing shoes." The laughing began again, and I felt extremely embarrassed, with such bad behaviour either side of me.

Fortunately, the bride arrived, and the service got underway. I personally was praying that it would all be over very soon, and I could make my get-away from this very tense situation.

The service proper was over, and the bride and groom departed to the vestry, for the signing of the marriage certificate. The vicar came to the front of the chancel, and said that whilst they were in the vestry, the choir would sing an anthem. Oh dear, I thought, this might be a bit awkward.

The four members of the choir came to the top of the chancel steps, and I nearly died when I saw that one of them was a little bald headed man. I knew instinctively that all hell would break out, but it was much worse than expected, when they struck up with the anthem. The singing was terrible, and I could feel vibrations coming along the seat, and Rob sitting next to me, was shaking in hysterics. It was the longest four minutes of my life, and despite being very annoyed with both Rob and Ian, I succumbed to the disgraceful laughter myself. I looked along the pew to my right, and everyone including Pat at the other end, was all creased up with the giggles.

It was one of those situations that you think will never end.

Financial Services

As explained earlier in this book, Rob worked for a number of years in the Financial Services business. During this time he was employed by several major insurance companies, and he has many wonderful stories to tell.

Whilst working for a major insurance group, the sales team were assembled in the regional office, planning their sales activity, and making customer appointments.

One of Rob's colleagues and good friend was Adrian, and a customer of his telephoned the office to query a recent statement, he'd received about his investment plan. The elderly gentleman on the phone said to Adrian. "Adrian, you know that investment plan that you sold me last year for £20 per month?" "Yes," said Adrian, "Well," said the elderly gentleman, "Can you come round and explain to my Missus, why after paying in a total of £240, my annual statement shows a current fund value of £157 cause I f****** can't." That was the kind of thing they had to deal with.

Incentive schemes

Whilst Rob was working for the same insurance group, they introduced a sales incentive scheme, which had a military theme.

The scheme was introduced by the branch manager Roger, who stood at the front of the sales team, dressed in a smart military uniform.

As you can imagine, the atmosphere was very tense, as the slightest thing would start them off with uncontrollable giggles. Rob had his mate Richard sat next to him, who was very prone to a lack of self-control.

Roger made the announcement that the first prize would be a two-week holiday to Thailand. At that stage, all was going well, and all the sales team seemed to be on their best behaviour. Then, someone near the front raised his hand and asked Roger if it would be possible to take children? A guy sat behind Rob then said, "That will all be taken care of when you get there!" The place erupted and Roger singled out Richard and asked him to leave the room.

Email protocols

During the monthly review meetings, the boss would lighten the mood by showing the sales team funny emails that he had received from colleagues; most of them involved some degree of nudity.

At one such meeting, the boss' big boss attended, purely as an observer, all part of the company's, team development strategy.

The meeting went fine, until the final item on the agenda, when the big boss made an announcement, that the company was aware of some individuals breaching the very strict policy regarding emails, and that any of them found doing so, would face strict disciplinary action. Whoops! Team boss, your secret's safe with us!!!

Procedures

The insurance industry is heavily regulated, and strict sales procedures need to be followed at all times. On one customer visit, Rob's boss accompanied him to observe him selling a pension plan to a lady customer. Rob carefully followed the long-winded procedures to the letter. All was going just fine, until one of the lady's work colleagues came over to offer some tea, and said to Rob, "There was none of this messing around last week, when you sold me my pension plan!"

Cats and laptops

One day, when Rob was working from home, his clingy and affectionate cat George, jumped up landing on Rob's laptop, and then fell off taking the computer keyboard with him. In a state of panic Rob telephoned the company IT department, and made up a story that his laptop must have been damaged, whilst in its carry bag.

He was hoping they would simply replace it, but instead, they asked him to courier the laptop back for repair. Rob was very worried that the IT people might smell a rat (or a cat) as to how the damage had occurred. A couple of days later, he received a message to contact the IT department immediately. Fearing the sack or some serious discipline, he contacted IT and they informed him that they had received the package, but then asked whether there was a laptop inside, when he dispatched it.

Obviously, the laptop had been stolen whilst in transit, which probably saved Rob's and George's bacon!!

Seminar presentations

According to Rob, performing at large seminars always had a fright element about it. He recalls one situation when he was on his feet presenting his introduction, and for some reason his confidence disappeared, leaving him speaking a load of verbal diarrhoea.

Sitting at the front, the course instructors had feed back forms, and following Rob's poor introduction, he observed a couple of them reach for their pens. Rob said, "For God's sake, don't fill in those feedback forms yet," to which they all laughed, and once again, Rob's humour had saved the day.

Laughing when you shouldn't

Rob tells a lovely story about the time when he was working for a major international insurance company. They had taken on four new starters including Rob, and he says they all had to endure the Monday morning meeting, where it was always inferred that if things didn't improve, their jobs would be on the line.

One of the new starters was a very smart young lady, who was experiencing great difficulty generating sales. She was always immaculately dressed, good with administration, always secured loads of appointments, talked a good job, but couldn't bring in the business. She was always punctual at these meetings, usually being the first of the four new starters to attend their Monday morning ritual.

One particular Monday, it was 09-15, and the dreaded meeting was in progress, but the young lady had not arrived. All of a sudden, the door burst open, and in she strides. She said she had been out driving the night before, when it had been very dark, and there was a cyclist. "Stop right there" said the manager, and Rob and his colleagues were asked to leave the room, whilst he spoke with the young lady in private.

Rob and his mate Colin went to make a brew, feeling somewhat relieved that so far into the meeting, there had been no rollicking forthcoming. As they were making the brew, there was a bit of a silence, and then Colin said "F*** me, she's killed someone." They both started laughing, not at the tragedy, simply because of the way Colin had said it. Next thing Colin says, "Oh heck, she's coming upstairs, stop laughing." She walked into the canteen, and two minutes later, Colin asked her what had happened. She went on to explain that she had witnessed a serious accident, the previous night.

In Rob's words "Sometimes in life, you think DON'T laugh, and it's not about the horrible story you've just heard, it's more to do with your mind saying, the worst thing I could do right now would be to laugh." Silence hung in the air, and Rob felt the need to say something profound. He thought "C'est La Vie" (That's Life in French) might be a good call, but saying it with a French accent wasn't, as he had no sooner said it than both he and Colin collapsed in laughter. The young lady broke into tears, and left the room. Twenty minutes later, Colin and Rob were summoned to the manager's office where upon, they received a real roasting from the manager, and a lecture about self-control!

'A' level studies

Rob took modular technology for one of his 'A' level qualifications, and part of the course involved a practical project. Ironically, as things were going to work out in a year or two's time, Rob decided to motorise a standard, push type, wheel chair.

To obtain greater knowledge about the construction of typical motorised wheel chairs, Rob asked if I would take a day's holiday, and drive him to an exhibition at the Crystal Palace in London. At the exhibition, Rob was able to ask lots of questions, and obtain contact details from manufactures, of motorised wheel chairs.

I was really impressed with him, because following the exhibition, he made contact with a wheel chair manufacturer in Birmingham, and after explaining what he was doing, he asked if they could help him obtain some second hand electric motors. Shortly afterwards, Rob asked me to drive him to this manufacturer, and the next available Saturday, we made our way to Birmingham.

I waited outside, and after a few minutes, Rob appeared carrying two motor driven geared units, ideal for his project.

He assembled the motors, whilst working at home in our garage. All was nearly complete, with chain drives to each wheel, and electronic controls. The project was almost finished, but he was experiencing some difficulty, wiring in the electric relays, to activate the motors. It was a soldering operation, and Rob being left handed, was finding it difficult to get the solder to adhere properly.

He asked me to assist, so we both went to the garage to get the soldering work completed. It was a winter's evening, and Rob was still wearing his smart Valley School sweater that had cost a lot of money. His mother had asked him to change his clothes beforehand, but he had not taken any notice.

I was working with the electric soldering iron, and like Rob, I was not finding it easy. I kept resting the electric soldering iron on top of the chest freezer, whilst it was getting hot. I kept smelling burn, but couldn't work out where it was coming from. Then Rob turned round and there was a damn great hole in the back of his school sweater, where it had obviously been in contact with the hot soldering iron. We were both horrified; we knew that we would be in deep trouble when Pat found out.

Typical of Rob and I; we both burst into fits of laughter, but eventually we had to go and face the music. You can imagine how she reacted, saying that the expensive sweater was ruined, and could not be mended.

Fortunately Rob passed his 'A' Modula Technology examination, getting very good marks for motorising the wheel chair.

Hospital visiting

Rob has always had a direct approach to life that was very evident on one occasion when he came to visit me in hospital. I had been feeling unwell, following a business trip to the USA. My doctor suspected Lyme disease, and I was admitted to Bassetlaw District Hospital, for tests and investigations,

I was 56 years of age at the time, and this was my first experience of hospitals, since my early childhood. I was very uptight about the whole thing, and worried about what the tests might involve.

I was admitted in the afternoon, and during the course of that evening, Rob came to visit. I spotted him strolling down the corridor carrying a plastic carrier bag. He approached my bed and handed me a pack of four cans of Guinness, plus a couple of magazines.

He then sat at me bedside and said, "Dad, if you're going to cock your clogs, can I please have your Gucci watch?"

This might seem more than a little insensitive, but typical of Rob, it was straight to the point.

I've had many a good titter about it since!!!

6

Recollections and Viewpoints

Rob's recollections of the accident

Although I have written this book from a family perspective, I wanted to include Rob's personal recollections of the accident, plus the period following his life saving surgery, when he lay in a coma, connected to a life support machine.

Rob had a premonition that something bad was going to happen to him, and that was the main reason why he had been putting so much effort into his bodybuilding exercises. He had not shared this fear with the family prior to the accident, but it was very clear in his mind, that something very unpleasant was on its way.

He remembers being out on the town with one of his mates Andy Sumpter, on the night of the injury, but has no recollections about the actual accident.

He cannot remember lying on the trolley at the Bassetlaw District Hospital, which having seen him first hand, is no surprise to me. No wonder I couldn't get any response from him, even though his eyes were wide open, he must have been completely unconscious.

The first thing Rob can recall following his emergency operation, is lying in intensive care with demonic like creatures, jumping off the wall at him. He describes them as Halloween characters, seeming half dream, and half reality.

Another dream, involved Rob's bed being in the middle of a forest, the same dream as in the film, 'An America Werewolf in London'. He also dreamt that an express train came speeding through the high dependency ward, and he couldn't understand why the nurse in attendance, took no notice of it whatsoever. None of these dreams were particularly scary, but their memory has remained with Rob after all these years.

I remember at some stage in Rob's recovery, visiting a customer of mine in Sheffield, who had suffered a similar head injury to Rob, and I was astonished when he described having the same dream about an express train speeding through his ward. Being an engineer, the guy described how he could smell the steam, and the oil, as well as hear all the associated noises, from such a splendid machine.

Rob's consultant explained that it was the opiate type drugs keeping him sedated and free of pain that had caused him to have these hallucinogenic dreams.

Apart from the dreams, the first real recollection from Rob was when Pat and Tracey were at his bedside, in the high dependency unit. He describes Pat standing at the left hand side of his bed, and Tracey stood on his right. He remembers his mother wearing a green blouse, and a tweed jacket. He also has clear recall of Pat's perfume, and that was the first thing he had smelt since his surgery. That perfume obviously had a major impact upon him, as he says he will never forget it.

He clearly remembers me going into the hospital one afternoon, to explain to him what had happened. We suspected, and quite rightly so, as Rob confirmed afterwards, that he had thought he might have been involved in a motoring accident.

When I informed him about his accident, whilst out in Worksop with his mate Andy Sumpter and what had transpired afterwards, Rob remembers showing the first signs of any emotion.

I questioned Rob further saying, do you have any additional memories from your time in a coma? This was his response:-

"I can't really say what a coma is like, because for a lot of the time, I was simply being kept alive, but I can assure you, for me, it wasn't a pleasant experience." He described it as a twisted reality and said, "Without sounding over the top, it's like walking a thin line between, living and dying." Rob understands that a lot of what he experienced was due to the drugs to control his brain from swelling, plus painkillers. He went on to say, "A coma was like a horrible nightmare, with short intervals of reality mixed in."

He clearly remembers communicating with his mother by blinking his eye, as well as squeezing Tracey's hand.

So what about how Rob felt having woken up from his coma, and lying there paralysed, and unable to speak?

He responded, "So how did I feel, lay in hospital bed with hardly the strength to keep my head balanced on my neck?" "Very very lucky indeed."

Rob went on, "I can best relate this to you by thinking about relative situations. If someone moved to a small terraced house from a six-bedroom property with a swimming pool, they would probably see this as a major step down. On the other hand, if someone had saved their hard earned money for many years, to put down a deposit on that same terraced house, then when they moved in, it would probably seem like their palace, same house but a different viewpoint. So me lay completely paralysed on a hospital bed, was not where I wished to be, but a far better place than where I had come from."

Rob describes two major positives from his memories of that time. Firstly, he still had his eyesight, and secondly, he had retained the ability to think and reason. Everything else could be rebuilt to something better, from where it was then. This was the overriding philosophy behind his positive attitude, and appreciation of escaping from the torment of lying in a coma.

He doesn't know when he came out of his coma, but thinks it was very similar to waking up from a deep sleep.

I have questioned Rob at length about his memories of what took place during the course of his hospitalisation, rehabilitation, and the period at home before returning to his work. I have incorporated many of these memories into the thread of the overall story, in the hope that the account of what took place is representative of several viewpoints, including that of Rob himself.

Coping with disability

Whilst Rob has handled his disability extremely well, I don't believe for one minute that it has been easy for him, and no doubt the problems regarding his physical limitations will continue.

A positive mental attitude, and a good sense of humour, are a major benefit, and fortunately Rob has an abundance of both these attributes.

He recalls a film entitled 'Born on the 4th July', in which a guy ends up in a wheel chair, following an injury in the Vietnam War. The guy is full of self-pity, and when an ex-army sergeant comes to visit, he shows no sympathy at all, and say's "Just get on with your life," or words to that effect. In Rob's words, "Now I didn't end up in a wheel chair or anything as major as that, therefore that sentiment probably seems a bit heavy, but I do strongly believe that if you're still here and enjoying life after a serious near fatal injury, then you are very lucky." "I may never be able to run again, so I don't dwell on that. Instead, I focus upon other things that are possible, and bring me enjoyment."

Rob remembers the attitude of certain people when he was in his wheel chair. He refers to a situation when Pat was pushing him along, and she came across a friend of hers.

Not looking at Rob, the friend addressed Pat and said, "How is he?" It's a well known fact that people in wheel chairs are often shunned, and I guess we've all heard the one about 'Does he take sugar?' Which must be very difficult to live with, if you are the person sitting in that wheel chair.

He describes his biggest fear post head injury was trying to be normal i.e. doing all the things that could be done prior to the accident. He says he wanted it so much, because it was hard to accept and be honest with others (particularly family) about his physical restrictions. Because of this, it was difficult for him to walk with people, especially when first meeting them, as his physical difficulties were very obvious, and he would tend to close-up, which made him struggle even more.

I asked Rob how he could pass on this same philosophy of positive attitude and fulfilment to others faced with similar disabilities. This was his response – *"It's a very simple concept, embrace everything you have, and work around things you don't.* He said, *"It's the easiest concept, but for me, I found great difficulty getting my head around it. For example, if I went on a journey with someone, and they parked the car, too far for me to walk I'd say, you know I'm disabled, so would you either park closer, or drop me at the door?" "Most people would accept this as a reasonable request, but for years I would find it difficult to ask, as I guess I'd see it as a sign of weakness. Disabled badges and mobility cars were there to help work around the things in life, which I could no longer do."*

"My second point is - don't stop doing the things you love within your restricted physical abilities." Fortunately for me, I never liked football or physical games but if I had, then watching would have to take precedence over playing those sports". "Also, for example I loved going to the pub for meeting friends and social interaction. I used to walk to the pub, and then move around several more, during the course of the evening. With that option no longer practical, I would go by taxi, and stay in the one pub rather than not go out at all."

"Cooking is another good example, I love to cook, but do get tired if I'm on my feet for any length of time. There are common sense ways to work around this, so if I need to chop vegetables for instance, I sit down and rest my aching legs.

Another difficulty to overcome is walking alongside others, worst of all when there is a group of people. My pace is slower than the average; therefore it is difficult to keep up. What tends to happen is that they speed off leaving you yards behind, feeling like a leper. There are two ways to overcome this situation, either say, "hey guys would you please slow down and wait for me," or alternatively, start an interesting conversation, to keep them at your pace. This may seen a very small point, but it is horrible when you are left trailing behind."

These mobility problems are likely to deteriorate as Rob gets older, and an example of this was experienced by Rob, following a holiday with his wife and children, in the summer of 2010. They stayed on a resort in Majorca, and Rob describes how people were strolling around not showing a care in the world. Not Rob, he was worried that he was going to struggle big time. He managed to get about for the first couple of days, but on the third day, his legs went into uncontrolled spasm. He simply couldn't walk very far at all, and the hot sunshine made matters worse.

He decided to hire a mobility scooter, and that restored his freedom of getting around. He had mixed feelings about the scooter, and felt he stood out like a sore thumb. He has an attractive wife, and to begin with, he was unhappy sat next to her on this mobility aid.

I have already referred to Rob's shoes in an earlier chapter but he has asked me to add some more detail. He says, "Please refer to shoes as following my head injury, they have been the bane of my life." "My feet are so over sensitive that I can trip very easily, and most ordinary casual shoes would send my feet into spasm." He describes shoe shopping as horrible, not caring about the style, he is far more concerned that the soles are sufficiently flexible to prevent his feet pushing down, and his toes turning over.

This problem is so bad that if he gets two pairs of shoes that are ok, changing from one to the other still causes spasms. He generally finds one pair that he can live with, until or course, they wear out.

Prejudice and self-confidence

Rob remembers going for a job interview a few years ago, and when the interviewer came to collect him from the waiting room, he realised Rob was trailing behind, and asked why? Rob explained that he had walking difficulties, following a serious head injury when he was eighteen years of age. Rob says, "He kept asking questions about my walking, so I became annoyed". The man said he needed to be sure that Rob was capable of doing the job. Rob goes on "This was a desk job, not a scaffolding job."

Rob believes in his heart of hearts, that the guy wasn't ok with disability, and he had similar instances, when attending other job interviews.

This is one reason why Rob went into the financial services industry, as there seemed to be far greater tolerance of employing individuals with disabilities. In Rob's words "It doesn't matter whether you have three heads, or you had been mining coal the week before, its how much you have sold that counts in that profession." This comment is probably a little extreme, but the financial services industry gave Rob an even playing field on which he could compete with his peers. Rob's physical disabilities still meant that he would always struggle to gain access to places, particularly if steps or staircases were involved, however I understand what he means regarding attitudes towards disability within that industry, because he always found colleagues very friendly and supportive, and it was Rob's sales results at the end of each month that was most important. It's a pity many more individuals, and organisations, are not demonstrating that commendable attitude towards disability.

On the subject of self-confidence, Rob describes how he initially developed a self-defeating attitude by thinking that an attractive young lady would never look at him. This meant that he was defeated even before he started.

He admits that he has prejudices just like everyone, we all have prejudices, but not all are admitted. He acknowledges that he would never date anyone obese, and that some people are put off by disability.

Rob says "It took me many years for the penny to drop, that personality and a sense of humour, will get you a long way."

Rob's final recommendation is to know your limitations. He says "work was becoming too much for me, and was causing direct physical affects on my body; it made me decide it was time to take things a bit easier."

Final comments

Rob sticks to his opinion that he has been very lucky following what may well have been a fatal head injury. I agree with this, but also make the point that he was very unlucky in the first place to have had the accident, and face such a severe set back in his early life. I remember discussing the nature of Rob's accident with the senior consultant responsible for Rob's care at the Royal Hallamshire Hospital. It was Rob's final meeting with the consultant, and when Rob described how the accident had happened; the consultant gave a beaming smile. When I questioned why he was smiling, he said that he did a similar thing to Rob, and fell following a few drinks, when out socialising with friends in Germany. Although the consultant severely banged his head, there was no internal damage. That's what I mean about Rob being unlucky, but I do admire his viewpoint and I'm convinced that it reflects his positive mental attitude, which has brought him back from those horrible dark days, now more twenty years ago.

As Rob's parents, Pat and I are very proud of our son, he has quite literally experienced a miraculous recovery and demonstrated what sheer determination, and fortitude can achieve. We are equally proud of our daughter Tracey, who was very special at the worst period following Rob's head injury, and her contribution to his remarkable recovery, will never be forgotten.

I do hope I have achieved a reasonable balance in writing this short book, as I feared it might appear that I have been dwelling in self-pity. Whilst Rob's situation was tough for each member of our immediate family, I don't wish to minimise the effects the shock had on our wider family plus many friends.

It has to be said that the person most affected by the accident was Rob, and the prime purpose behind this biographical account of his story, was to pay tribute to the man himself, for the manner in which he coped with the trauma of the injury, and then how he applied himself, showing immense courage and a positive attitude, that greatly assisted him through his long journey back.

Lightning Source UK Ltd.
Milton Keynes UK
178424UK00001B/37/P